Your Key to
Good Health

Your Key to
Good Health
Unlocking the Power of Your
Lymphatic System

Elaine Hruska

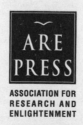

ASSOCIATION FOR
RESEARCH AND
ENLIGHTENMENT

A.R.E. Press • Virginia Beach • Virginia

ISBN 978-0-87604-570-1 (trade pbk.)

The contents of this publication are intended for educational and informative use only. They are not to be considered directive nor as a guide to self-diagnosis or self-treatment. Before embarking on any therapeutic regimen, it is absolutely essential that you consult with and obtain the approval of your personal physician or health care provider.

Cover illustration by artist Sebastian Kaulitzki

CONTENTS

INTRODUCTION

Why a book on lymph? This rather unexplored and until lately poorly un-derstood system of the physical body has remained mysterious and largely ignored for centuries. Even in the 1930s, when Edgar Cayce was busy carrying on his life's work of giving readings, the lymphatic system was considered off-limits not only for physicians but also for physical therapists and mas-sage practitioners. If clients or patients, for example, presented themselves with swollen lymph nodes in their necks, the therapist was taught to refrain from massaging or even touching the area. It was believed or thought by the medical community that palpating the swollen nodes or surrounding areas would spread bacteria and viruses, thus increasing infection throughout the body of the client and, as a result, worsening the condition. Because of this mistaken belief and taboo plus lack of knowledge, the lymphatic system was to a great extent disregarded by health care professionals and therapists who did not want to create additional sickness in their clients. Until recently it was common for children with swollen neck nodes or tonsils to have them surgi-cally removed. Spleens and appendixes were likewise removed, their value as a component of the body's defense system not being discovered until later.

That interest and concern in this topic have gradually increased during this present time period (when individuals are choosing and demanding a more holistic approach and are willing to shoulder some responsibility for the onset of their illness) is also demonstrated by the amount of material covered in anatomy and physiology texts. In the mid-1980s, when I attended massage school, the textbook devoted eighteen pages to a chapter entitled "The Lymphatic System"; however, seven of those pages contained full–page illustrations. Some years later, the lymphatic system merited thirty–seven pages with half– or full–page illustrations and charts covering twelve of those pages. Why this shift in the amount of material and information? Not only is the description of lymph vessels more detailed, but the effect of that system upon the body is better understood and acknowledged. Yet the average person, as represented by those who come for services to the A.R.E. Health Center and Spa, has little knowledge or conception of what the lymph consists of or how the system operates. Unless clients have encountered a specific health problem (sometimes after surgery or an injury) of edema (swelling), they may not be aware of the condition of their lymphatic system or even pay much attention to it.

The physical readings of Edgar Cayce, in a number of instances way ahead of the times, have a lot to say about lymph and its effect on disease and health. There are, in fact, a little over three thousand references or mentions of lymph and lymphatic vessels in the total body of text. Considering that 9,541 physical readings exist, references to the lymphatic system, then, constitute nearly one–third of occurrences throughout these readings. That is quite an "honorable mention" when one realizes how scant attention was being paid to this system at the time the readings were being given, as well as little recognition and understanding of its function and operation.

One exception to this, in addition to Cayce, was a contemporary of Cayce's, Dr. Andrew Taylor ("A.T.") Still (1828–1917), who is considered the founder of osteopathy. In a biography, *The Lengthening Shadow of Dr. Andrew Taylor Still*, written by one of his students, Arthur Grant Hildreth (also an osteopath), is a description of how Dr. Still approached each patient of his, attempting to diagnose and figure out what was occurring in each one's physical body. After going through various organs and systems in the body—much like Cayce did in his trance physical readings—and then describing the function of the arterial and venous systems, Still added:

There is still a third and most important system of vessels which accompanies the arteries and veins throughout the body. This is known as the lymphatic system. It supplies the serous fluid in which the tissue cells are bathed. It has to do with the mechanism of nutrition, absorption, and the protection of cells from harmful poisons and bacteria. p. 183

This succinct summary of what Still considered the job of the lymphatic system is mirrored as well in Cayce's readings. In this book an attempt will be made to present Cayce's perspective on the lymph, including the numerous health conditions resulting from its poor functioning plus helpful hints from the readings and other sources on how to alleviate and reverse these conditions. With the increase in concern and interest nowadays in the body's immune system, along with continuing observation and study of autoimmune diseases (in which the immune system reacts against the body's own tissues), it becomes imperative to learn how we can function more optimally and not take for granted the role the lymphatic system plays in helping us achieve stability and balance as well as relief from some of its destructive symptoms. We will no doubt be amazed and surprised at the importance of the lymphatic system in maintaining our overall health and well-being. It is hoped that these goals will be achieved in the content of this present book.

Note to the Reader: The Edgar Cayce readings are catalogued numerically. Each recipient of a reading was assigned a number to provide anonymity. The first set of numbers refers to the individual or group who received the reading; the second set represents its place in a sequence. For example, in reading 294-3, "294" stands for the person's name, while "-3" means this was the third reading given for that individual.

When the readings were computerized, the body of the reading was referred to as the "text." Any notes, letters, background information, related articles, and so on, were also placed with the reading. In terms of style, R stands for reports and B stands for background. To locate this information easier, these letters are used. For example, 202-1, R-5 means that in reading 202-1 under reports (R), item number 5, can be found that particular quote.

The language of the readings can be quite challenging. Rather than try to paraphrase, I felt it was better to quote the text verbatim. Oftentimes reading the quote several times may be required to grasp its meaning.

The readings were given for individuals, yet they carry a universality of content. With the physical readings, however, it is important that the information not be used for self-diagnosis or self-treatment. Any medical problems need the supervision and advice of a health care professional.

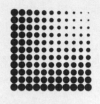

CHAPTER ONE
· · · · · · · · · · ·

The Cayce Health Readings:
A Brief Overview

Edgar Cayce, who lived from 1877 to 1945, was a remarkable individual. For most of his adult life he gave what are called "readings," discourses for people who requested information on a variety of topics. He did all this in a sleeplike state; that is, he appeared to be asleep, yet could respond to questions posed to him, giving replies that far exceeded what he knew consciously. While the accuracy of this information is largely still being tested, the suggestions and recommendations—though given for a specific individual who asked for the reading—have proven helpful to many others with similar situations or complaints. Called the father of the modern–day holistic health movement in America because of the nature of his discourses, Cayce gave thousands of readings, more than fourteen thousand of which are housed in the A.R.E. Library in Virginia Beach, Virginia, and are available for study and inspection by the public. Of these readings, 9,541, or about 67 percent of the total, are categorized as physical readings, since they deal with the health concerns of those seeking guidance for their ailments. It's fairly safe to state that, when the recipient of the reading followed through with the recommendations contained in it, the results were generally successful. Reports filed along with the reading attested to these outcomes; unfortunately, for a number of cases no follow-up information was forthcoming: the client did not communicate any results or did not return questionnaires. Some followed the suggestions in part or did not attempt the therapies at all. While such outcomes might be frustrating to those wishing proof of their validity, enough information exists to help confirm the accuracy of the diagnoses as well as the helpfulness of the recommended treatments.

FOLLOWING A HEALTH READING

What if an individual today who has a particular health concern would like to attempt a holistic approach as Cayce advocated? What could he or she do about following Cayce's advice? Several options are open:

1.   Read all the readings that cover your particular ailment. A listing of many different diseases and physical concerns are found in the Circulating File Index (medical section). These individual Files can be purchased or ordered on loan; they are small booklets that contain most of the readings on a particular ailment. Decide from this compilation which readings and/or treatments you'd like to follow.

2.   Check out or purchase a Research Bulletin. Each one documents a disease along with a commentary, representative readings, and a statistical abstract classifying causes and treatments of the disease. While physical topics for these Bulletins are limited, they do offer the most often recommended remedies for each ailment along with a general overview of the problem.

3.   Individual Research Protocols—binders of standardized health packages on nearly fifty specific illnesses—can be purchased through the A.R.E. These explain in layperson's terms the process used in following the recommendations suggested in the readings for each ailment. You are also invited to participate in a research project on remedies that were recommended for that particular disease.

4.   A suggestion offered by Gladys Davis Turner, Cayce's longtime secretary, was to examine all of the readings specific to your condition.

Then choose one reading that matches or resembles most closely your current physical condition, your particular symptoms, same sex, same age or close to your age, and so forth, and follow the suggestions Cayce gave for that person.

While medical terminology has changed since Cayce's day and new designations of diseases have arisen, it may be more difficult to locate in the readings particular symptoms or conditions that are prevalent today. Yet, through ongoing study and research into the health readings, updates are continuously being made and noted, with the idea of being more serviceable to the individual seeker.

ORIGIN OF INFORMATION

An important question—especially when dealing with psychic readings—is, Where is the information coming from? When we take the time, energy—and money!—to seek answers beyond and outside of ourselves, it is imperative that we question the source of the information. A unique aspect of the body of Cayce's material is the set of readings called the Work Readings, the 254 series, which was devoted to questions and comments on just what to do with or how to develop this material so that it would be beneficial and helpful to others. One such reading in this series described the seeker's part in making the effort to obtain health information: "When an individual seeks for personal or bodily aid, it is part and parcel of that individual and [the information] is read by and through the real desire of the seeker." (254-95) This places a degree of responsibility on the part of the recipient as to what is "the real desire," what is the purpose for the request, why is one *really* asking for this reading. Then, according to this excerpt, the material that is forthcoming from the psychic who is dispensing the information will be colored by the recipient's motives and desires. The resultant reading would need to be studied and analyzed with these purposes in mind.

While a number of sources were given for the body of Cayce's readings—for example, for life readings the information was obtained from the Book of Life, or the Akashic Records, of that particular individual—the health information was fairly specific regarding the origin. As stated in the above excerpt, the information "is part and parcel of that individual" seeking. Does this mean that we *do* know the source or origin of our illness? That it is indeed a part of us already? Which part? If this information is stored within us, then we already know what has created our sickness—better even perhaps than any psychic—and we also know what route we need to take to return to better health. Another reading alludes to this same concept: "From any subconscious mind information may be obtained . . . as we see a mirror reflecting direct that which is before it." (3744–3)

According to a number of sources, the subconscious mind is like a storehouse of memories that have been forgotten, where suppressed thoughts and ideas remain hidden, where knowledge not needed is held in abeyance, and maybe even details of former incarnations are shelved. Through the process of giving a reading, Cayce's conscious mind was laid aside (as if he were asleep), and his subconscious mind became activated, attuning itself "with the purpose of the seeker" (294–202), to give the information based upon the suggestion offered at the beginning of the reading itself. Cayce, as the channel for this work, already prepared himself through prayer and meditation and by setting an ideal of service, and the ones requesting the reading were to "attune themselves to that promise which was made to this entity, Edgar Cayce." (294–202)

The "promise" mentioned here refers to an event from Cayce's boyhood, as recounted in several biographies. When he was about twelve years old, Edgar had an encounter with an angelic presence as he was reading his Bible. The angel asked him what he would like most of all, and he replied, "To be helpful to others, especially children when they are sick." Evidently pleased with this selfless reply, the angel promised fulfillment of his wish. Those tens of thousands of individuals who obtained readings from Cayce all became beneficiaries of this generous legacy.

If one's own subconscious mind is the real origin of information for one's physical ailments, the people who requested readings from Cayce were, in essence, asking him to "read their minds." In his altered state, Cayce could do this simply and easily, acting upon the suggestion that was read aloud to him by the conductor of the reading (usually his wife, Gertrude). The subsequent discourse, taken down in shorthand by his secretary, most often Gladys Davis Turner, offered a detailed analysis of one's physical condition plus a treatment protocol to follow.

A TYPICAL PHYSICAL READING

For a health reading, the usual suggestion followed this formula, which over a period of time was refined to these words:

> You have the body of [individual's name] before you, who is in [city and street address given]. You will go over this body carefully, examine it thoroughly, and tell me the conditions you find at the present time, giving the cause of the existing conditions, also the treatment for the cure and relief of this body. You will speak distinctly at a normal rate of speech, answering the questions as I ask them.

After a pause, Cayce would usually begin, "Yes, we have the body here . . . " Often referring to himself in the plural—the editorial "we"—Cayce seemed to feel in close proximity to the seeker, as if he or she were right next to him, present in the room with him. Often this was not the case. The individual could be thousands of miles from Virginia Beach, where Cayce gave most of his readings. Yet, in this psychic realm, distance was no hindrance, no barrier.

Next, Cayce usually made some opening remarks, covering the general physical conditions that he found in the body, such as:

> Now, we find the body is very good in many respects. There are those conditions rather of which the body should be warned, and of some corrections that should be made, that there might be better functioning throughout the system, for the deficiency in the more normal functioning lies in the glands of the body. Now, these, then, are the conditions, physical, as we find in this body. First . . .

Following this general introduction came a more detailed description of the body from the standpoint of the blood supply, the nerve system, and the condition of the organs involved. In the typed copy of the reading, these divisions were sometimes capitalized, as if they were headers, delineating major sections in the description of the physical body. Using terms and language that seem a bit archaic today, the Cayce source pinpointed the cause of the problem, explained what was occurring physiologically, and pointed out the consequences on different areas of the body—in effect, a comprehensive view of the inner workings of the particular physical body along with side comments sometimes regarding attitudes to be either adopted or changed. The overall picture was of an interconnected system, or web, with one part dependent and affected by another, all parts working together in a marvelous whole.

This analysis in itself would be priceless—a thorough review of just what was happening inside one's self. Yet there was more: an itemized, often step-by-step procedure outlining treatments to be undertaken. So the recipient was not merely left in the lurch with only a diagnosis, but the remedies were at hand for dealing with the imbalance. The suggestions covered a wide range of fields of study—herbs, spinal manipulations, homeopathy, surgery, hydrotherapy, diet, tonics, appliances—using a rather comprehensive, all-inclusive model for healing. Included with the detailed instructions were often words of hope and encouragement, sometimes near the conclusion of the discourse, that if the suggestions were followed, health and healing were assured.

Then the lengthy description ended, and the typical phrase "Ready for questions" announced a shift in focus. Immediately a question-and-answer period followed, usually with questions that had been submitted earlier by the recipient, which Cayce hardly ever looked at. Yet often it was discovered that the questions had already been answered within the text of the reading. Some questions were delivered spontaneously, asking for explanations on sections of the reading that were not quite clear to the recipient or on topics not addressed in the reading. Complaints that were still uppermost in importance were addressed; however, the reply might be given that following the treatments would take care of the problem.

When the questions were completed, the discourse ended with a statement similar to "We are through for the present." The whole process may have taken a few minutes to an hour, depending upon the length of the reading. The suggestion was then given by the conductor to Edgar Cayce to awaken, much like coming out of a hypnosis session.

Usually, the words were not written down in the text of the reading, as it was largely the same formula given from one reading to the next. The recipient now had some material with which to work and could choose more wisely and carefully the course of treatment to follow.

CONCLUSION

What must it have been like to receive a physical reading from Edgar Cayce? A number of recipients were desperate, searching for the cause of and a solution to their crisis. They had already traveled the medical route, seeing one professional after another. When they obtained their reading through the mail, they were often filled with hope. They had some answers, something positive to work with, a plan to follow. No doubt, most of them had no inkling that years later others would be studying the advice and guidance given them, also hoping for solutions or clues to their dilemmas. Through today's technology the readings have become more accessible, so this ongoing search continues, accompanied by further study and research to make it more practical and beneficial for others.

Before discussing Cayce's health readings concerning the lymphatic system, we will present in the next chapter some information on the basics of this system to help you, the reader, better understand and comprehend the workings of this valuable function in the human body.

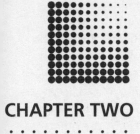

CHAPTER TWO
. . . .

Basics of the Lymphatic System: Lymph 101

We may become ill because of an outbreak of the "common cold," with its accompanying runny nose, sore throat, and swollen neck nodes. Or a sinus infection hits us with its usual postnasal drip. A scratch or cut becomes infected, then reddens and swells. Upon awakening one morning, we might feel sluggish, barely able to get out of bed, and notice swelling of our hands or ankles. All of these symptoms are indications or disturbances arising from the functioning—or lack of proper functioning—of our lymphatic system. They offer us clues that this system is draining poorly or is moving sluggishly. Often upper respiratory infections (such as sinusitis or tonsillitis) or lower respiratory infections (such as pneumonia or bronchitis) are indicative of a lymph drainage problem. Poor circulation, signified by cold hands or feet or numbness and tingling, may also be the result of sluggish lymphatic drainage.

What constitutes the lymphatic system, and what is its function? We may all be familiar with the circulatory, nervous, digestive, reproductive, and excretory systems from our elementary and high school science classes. They are considered the five main divisions through which our body functions and operates and carries on its work. But where does the lymphatic system belong in our body's complex array of working parts?

The lymphatic system is actually a specialized component of our circulatory system, which generally consists of veins, arteries, and capillaries through which blood is pumped by action of the heart. The lymph fluid, like blood, also moves throughout the body and serves as a unique transportation vehicle; it returns substances, such as proteins, fats, dead cells, and tissue fluids, to the general circulation. It's an accessory route, collecting the fluid that flows from the spaces in between the cells (interstitial fluid) and eventually depositing it into the bloodstream. Unlike the blood, however, there is no muscular pumping organ like the heart to force the fluid through the body, yet by various means this fluid does move along steadily and slowly between the cells and throughout its vessels. As a rule of thumb, the lymphatic and capillary (blood) networks lie side by side, broadly parallel and in close proximity to each other, yet they remain separate and independent of the other.

One very important function of the lymphatic system is its ability to carry away from the tissue spaces proteins and large particulate matter, neither of which can be placed directly into the blood capillary. You might think, so what? What's so fantastic about moving these substances from the fluid between the cells into the bloodstream? However, the removal of proteins from these spaces is an absolutely essential function, for without it we would die within close to twenty-four hours. Take note of this quote from Guyton's *Anatomy and Physiology*:

> The single most important function of the lymphatics is to return proteins to the circulation when they leak out of the blood capillaries. Some of the pores in the capillaries are so large that small amounts of proteins leak continuously, amounting each day to approximately one-half of the total protein in the circulation. If these proteins were not returned to the circulation, the person's plasma colloid osmotic pressure [pressure that moves fluid into the capillary] would fall so low and he would lose so much blood volume into the interstitial spaces that he would die within twelve to twenty-four hours. Furthermore, no other

means is available by which proteins can return to the circulation except
by way of the lymphatics. p. 511

So if it were not for this ongoing removal of proteins, life could no
longer continue. The exchange of fluids would be so abnormal that we
would cease to exist. As stated in the quote, no other route exists in our
bodies except the lymphatics to return these excess proteins to the circulatory system. Hence, no other function of the lymphatic system can
even approach this highly important, life-sustaining role.

MAIN PARTS OF THE SYSTEM

Structurally, the lymphatic system is composed of lymph, lymphatic
vessels, lymph nodes, Peyer's patches, and lymphatic organs. (See Fig. 1.)
Serving as a defense against infection, the lymphatic system plays an
important role in the body's immunologic response as well as helps to
maintain a balance of fluids in the body. A network of lymph nodes
clustered in groups and connected by lymphatic vessels make up part
of this vast system, which resembles a tree with its main trunk located
at the center of the body, its branches reaching out with smaller and
smaller twigs, and its foliage covering most of the human body. Or it
can be said to resemble an extensive subway system, with its many
tubes and tunnels running throughout the body. (See Fig. 2.)

Looking more carefully at each component of the lymphatic system,
mentioned above, we have the following descriptions:

Lymph is a clear, watery-appearing fluid, originating in the connective
tissue spaces of the body. It is still a mystery, however, exactly how it is
formed. The fluid is referred to as *lymph* once it enters the initial lymph
capillaries and is carried through the *lymphatic vessels* (lymphatics) to
lymph nodes, to ducts and trunks, then to the venous system, eventually
reaching the heart. Interstitial fluid, the watery substance found in between the cells, is formed by components of blood plasma that have
filtered through the blood capillary walls. Yet lymph and interstitial
fluid are similar: the former is located within lymphatic vessels and
lymphatic tissue, while the latter is found in between the cells.

Lymphatic vessels begin as closed-end structures called lymphatic

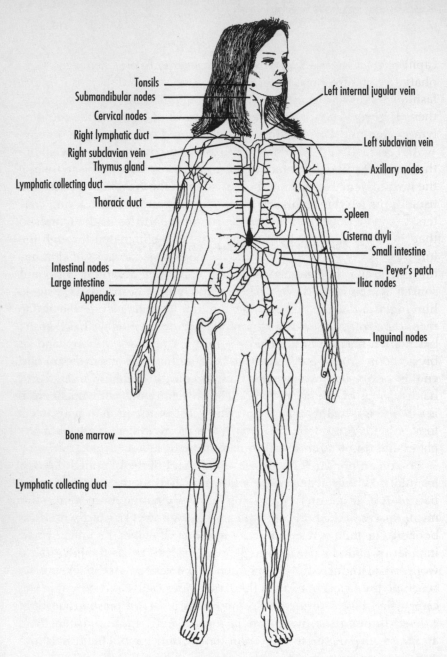

Figure 1
Principal components of the lymphatic system

Drawing by Evan Van Auken

capillaries. Just as smaller blood capillaries eventually form veins, lymphatic capillaries unite to form larger and larger tubes. In a similar fashion, but in reverse, a large tree trunk divides into smaller branches, then into even smaller twigs. As noted above, these vessels (also called lymphatics) route the lymph fluid on its way to the heart.

At various intervals, like subway stations, the lymph fluid flows through **lymph nodes,** oval or bean–shaped structures located along the length of the lymphatic vessels. Scattered throughout the body and usually clustered in groups, they act as purification and filtering centers, breaking down and destroying harmful particles in the lymph so that they can be flushed out of the body and eliminated through the lungs, skin, kidneys, and intestines, the body's main organs of elimination. We usually become aware of them when they become swollen and somewhat achy and painful. There can be from four hundred to seven hundred nodes in the human body, nearly half of them in the abdomen; the others are located in the neck region, armpits (axillae), groin, behind the knees (popliteal area), in the bend of the elbows, and in breast tissue. Flowing in one direction, lymph enters the nodes at one end and exits at another, in the process being cleansed of foreign and harmful substances. As it travels through the nodes, the flow of lymph is usually slowed, allowing time for this cleansing and filtering process to take place. The nodes are also the site of maturation for some lymphocytes, a type of white blood cell important to the body's defense system.

Peyer's patches are large specialized collections of lymphoid tissue located in the small intestine, particularly in the ileum. They were named after Johann K. Peyer (1653–1712), a Swiss anatomist, and are mentioned in over sixty readings by Cayce. Bacteria, which enter the body through the mouth, eventually penetrate into the wall of the small intestine, where they multiply in the area of the Peyer's patches. After a week or two, the bacteria enter the bloodstream. The Cayce readings concur with this function, recognizing this area as the place where poisons can be absorbed into the system. (More about this structure in chapter 5.)

Lastly, we have the **lymphatic organs:** tonsils, thymus, spleen, liver, appendix, and bone marrow. They, too, help the body fight infection, each in its own unique way.

The **tonsils** are located at the back of the mouth, at either side of the

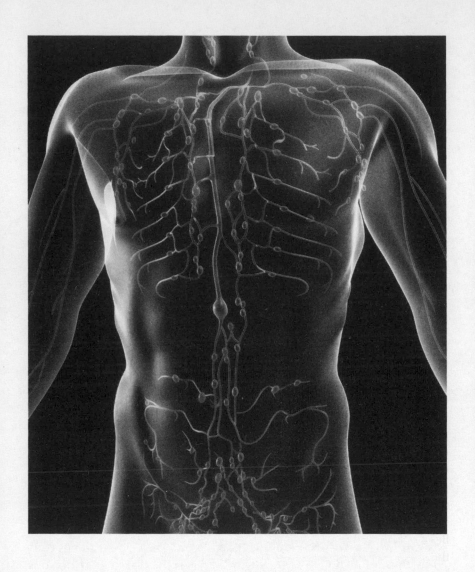

Figure 2
The lymphatic vessels, larger lymphatic trunks, and lymph nodes

throat. They assist in trapping and destroying microorganisms and keeping infections away from the lungs. During childhood, around ages six or seven, they are the largest in size but gradually shrink through-out one's life. They are removed usually in cases where recurrent at-tacks of tonsillitis (inflammation and swelling of the tonsils) may interfere with the child's breathing, swallowing, or general health, but—aside from these instances—the operation is usually not necessary and only performed as a last resort.

In the long unrecognized *thymus,* a small gland near the heart, the cells of the immune system learn to differentiate self from non–self. When the immune system starts developing in the fetus, stem cells mi-grate to the thymus. Here they develop into T lymphocytes, white blood cells which help protect against viral infections as well as detect and destroy some cancer cells. (When these T lymphocytes lose their ability to differentiate self from non–self, autoimmune disease may result.) That it plays a critical part in the body's defense against infection was not well known until the 1960s. Largest in size at puberty, the gland gradu-ally shrinks and eventually atrophies when the person is much older, its lymphatic tissue replaced by fat, perhaps completing most of its es-sential work early in childhood. Despite this atrophy, however, some T cells continue to proliferate in the thymus throughout one's lifetime.

About the size of a fist, the *spleen,* which is the largest mass of lym-phatic tissue in the body, is located in the upper left part of the abdomi-nal cavity, just under the rib cage. Its function is to produce, monitor, store, and destroy blood cells. Its spongelike tissue is of two types: white pulp, which is part of the infection–fighting (immune) system and where some lymphocytes are produced, and red pulp, which removes un-wanted material from the blood, especially defective red blood cells. Before birth, red blood cells are formed here, and in the normal adult the spleen serves as a reservoir for blood. If it is surgically removed, the body loses some of its ability to produce protective antibodies and to extract unwanted substances from the blood, thus lessening one's abil-ity to fight infection. However, other organs, especially the liver, will compensate for this loss and take up the infection–fighting job.

One of the largest organs in the body, the *liver* is also one of the most important. Similar to a chemical processing plant, it performs a variety of vital functions: production of cholesterol and bile; manufacturing of proteins; storage of iron, glycogen, and vitamins; removal of poisons and waste products from the blood; and conversion of waste to urea. It is also a main component of the digestive system, though it lies outside of the digestive tract. Because it filters and destroys bacteria and helps detoxify the body, some texts (for example, *The Merck Manual*) list it as part of the lymphatic system as well. Located in the upper right section of the abdomen behind the lower ribs, it is dark red in color and one of the most versatile organs in our body.

The **appendix,** also called vermiform appendix, is a small, finger-shaped, wormlike tube that projects from the ascending colon (on the right side of the abdomen) of the large intestine at its junction with the small intestine. Because it is chiefly lymphatic tissue, an infection anywhere in the body that also produces enlarged lymph nodes can increase its glandular tissue, eventually causing inflammation and infection. Unless the body's defenses overcome the infection, the appendix may have to be removed before it ruptures, leading to peritonitis, a serious and dangerous condition. Sometimes considered a rather useless structure, it is often routinely removed by surgery because of its potential for this painful and serious inflammation.

Red blood cells, white blood cells, and platelets are produced in the **bone marrow,** which is the innermost portion of the bone and shaped like a hollow cavity. In response to infection, the bone marrow produces and releases more white blood cells, the body's major mechanism for fighting infections. When blood cells for some reason show abnormalities, a bone marrow examination is often used to determine the cause. Disorders of bone marrow include diseases in which either too many or too few blood cells are produced.

From this brief overview of the main components of the lymphatic system, we may get a sense of the important role it plays in our body's overall health and well-being. Just the extent and pervasiveness of this system, affecting a wide range of tissues, organs, and vessels, may give us a clue to the necessity of caring for it and keeping it working in an optimal fashion.

Here follow a few more points regarding the composition of the lymphatic system:

Analogous to the tree trunk, mentioned earlier as a visual description, are two large, main lymphatic vessels: the **thoracic duct** and the **right lymphatic duct** (the latter actually comprises three collecting ducts). These structures, located roughly in the center of the thorax, are the principal channels through which lymph passes into the venous blood. (See Fig. 1.) They serve as receivers of the lymph from the whole body: lymph from the body's upper right quadrant drains into the right lymphatic duct (and then into the right subclavian vein), while lymph from the rest of the body drains into the thoracic duct (and then into the left subclavian vein). (See Fig. 3.) As their names indicate, the subclavian veins are located underneath the right and left clavicles (collarbones) in the upper chest area. Thus, the important function of lymphatic vessels is now fulfilled: to return "leaked" plasma proteins and fluid, arising from the spaces between the cells and flowing through the lymphatics, and finally deposit them in the bloodstream.

Schematically, the flow of fluid, then, may be represented in this manner (the words in parentheses give the name of the fluid in those vessels): arteries (blood plasma) ➜ blood capillaries ➜ interstitial spaces (interstitial fluid) ➜ lymphatic capillaries (lymph) ➜ lymphatic vessels ➜ lymph nodes ➜ lymphatic trunks ➜ lymphatic ducts ➜ subclavian veins (blood plasma). This "flow chart" represents the origins of the fluid: one that "leaks" from or seeps out of the blood (arteries) plus the fluid that fills the spaces between the cells (interstitial fluid). This excess fluid, about three liters per day, is collected and drains, then, into lymphatic capillaries, where it becomes lymph; it ultimately enters into the venous blood through the subclavian veins. In truth, the lymphatic system is a second circulatory system, carrying lymph instead of blood, and traveling through various lymphatic vessels, which resemble capillaries and veins, on its way back to the heart. Its chief function is to help drain the excess fluid from the interstitial area and to pick up proteins that may have leaked out of the capillaries.

ORIGIN AND HISTORY OF LYMPH

We exist within our bodies in a wet world, water comprising 70–80 percent of our being. Flowing between all the cells, interstitial fluid

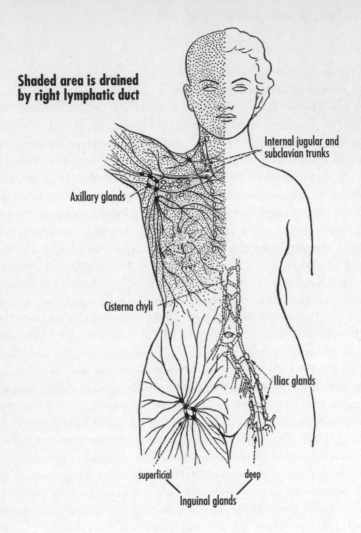

Shaded area is drained by right lymphatic duct

Internal jugular and subclavian trunks

Axillary glands

Cisterna chyli

Iliac glands

superficial

deep

Inguinal glands

Figure 3
Drainage of lymphatic fluid

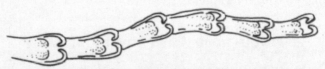

Figure 4
Lymphatic capillaries and vessel wall musculature.

bathes these cells with life–giving substances. Its clear, colorless liquid carries such microscopic particles as white blood cells, proteins, and other substances vital to the life of the cell. Blood capillaries also exude fluid into tissues, but not all this fluid returns to the blood, thus creating an accumulation, or excess, of tissue fluid. Collecting this excess fluid from between the cells and eventually returning it to the body's circulation is the purpose for this vast lymphatic network, with its miles of tubes and channels of interconnected vessels. When too much of the interstitial fluid accumulates, the lymphatic vessels, as stated previously, channel it through a series of closed–end tubules. Now it is called lymph, a word derived from the Latin *lympha*, meaning "clear water" or "spring water."

According to *Webster's New World Dictionary* (3rd college edition), the word *lymph* is also influenced etymologically by the Greek *nymphē*, our English word *nymph*. In Roman and Greek mythology, nymphs were a group of minor nature goddesses, usually represented as young and beautiful, who inhabited rivers, springs, seas, or lakes: that is, places of clear water. The word *limpid*, with similar origin, means "perfectly clear; transparent; not cloudy or turbid."

Owing to its transparent quality, lymph is difficult to see during dissections, so its discovery as part of an integrated system in the body developed slowly over time and arrived late on the medical scene.

Some ancient civilizations—such as China, India, and Egypt—had elementary notions of a "white blood," possibly referring to the milky, intestinal lymph fluid that follows digestion of a fatty meal. Traditional Chinese medicine speaks of a water element connected with the bladder and kidney meridians; it differentiated between liquids of the body and blood. Ancient India's Ayurvedic medicine had knowledge of "interstitial liquid," which represented one of the seven systems of the body. According to the ancient Egyptians, the heart contained liquid; vessels existed that transported organic substances throughout the body.

The Greek physician Hippocrates (c. 460–c. 377 B.C.), often referred to as the Father of Medicine, noted and recognized a milky–white material being drained from the intestines and conjectured that this substance resulted from digested fatty material. This was later shown to be an accurate assessment. He was the first to use the word *chyle* (a milky fluid formed in the small intestine, composed of lymph and emulsified fats) and also listed a "lymphatic (phlegmatic) temperament" as one of the four main temperaments of the human being. Other ancient physicians did not clearly differentiate blood from lymph, yet they traced the lymph channels in the same geographic pattern as veins (vessels which return blood back to the heart). The actual pathway of these lymph vessels flowing into the bloodstream was not properly mapped until centuries later.

Aristotle (384–322 B.C.) spoke about structures with transparent fluid, while Herophilus (335–280 B.C.) noted the presence of mesenteric lymph nodes and "milky veins" (lacteals). During the course of the centuries following further observations and speculations, there was a surge in the seventeenth century that offered more insights and clarity into the nature of the lymphatic system. Just a few years before William Harvey (1578–1657) presented the physiology of the cardiovascular system in his published works (1628), Gasparo Asselli (1581–1626) noted the "white and milky veins" of a dog in 1622, the first documented discovery of the lymphatic vessels. In 1653 Johann Vesling (1598–1649) followed with the first illustrations of human lymphatics, but it was Olof Rudbeck (1630–1708), a Swedish anatomist and "Renaissance man," who first recognized the lymphatic system as a complete system and as a part of the circulation. Using the ligature technique, he dissected more than four hundred animals to substantiate his ideas. Other scientists followed and built upon these discoveries and observations with their own theories of the flow of lymph and its function and role in the human body.

THE FLOW OF LYMPH

If the lymphatic system, as mentioned near the beginning of this chapter, does not have a muscular pumping organ (like the circulatory system does with the heart), how does the fluid get passed along through the various vessels and ducts? As an accessory route, this system does serve a unique transport function in that it returns tissue fluid, proteins, fats, and other substances to the general circulation. Yet there are differences from the true circulation of blood (as seen in the makeup of our cardiovascular system) to the flow of lymph. Unlike vessels in the blood vascular system, lymphatic vessels form only half a circuit, that is, they do not form a closed ring: there is not a continuous pathway with a "beginning" and an "end," like the route of blood in its flow to and from the heart. Lymphatic vessels begin blindly in the intercellular spaces of the soft tissues of the body, collect the excess fluid there, finally draining it into the blood vascular venous system, and returning it to the heart.

The two systems, though, closely parallel each other and work in conjunction with each other. In the skin, lymphatic vessels lie in the subcutaneous tissue (under the skin) and generally follow veins, while lymphatic vessels of the viscera (organs) generally follow arteries, forming plexuses (networks) around them. To understand more clearly how the lymph flows throughout the body, it is helpful to examine the composition and structure of lymphatic capillaries, which constitute the beginning of lymphatic vessels.

All lymphatic vessels originate as lymphatic capillaries (also known as initial lymph vessels), tiny structures located in the spaces between the cells. Resembling a vast network of vessels, they form a fine mesh covering most of the body. Because their diameters are larger than blood capillaries, large substances that cannot be absorbed into a blood capillary (such as proteins) can be removed from the interstitial spaces and eventually returned to the blood.

Lymphatic capillaries have a unique structure that permits interstitial fluid to flow into them but not out. The ends of the endothelial cells that make up the inner walls of the capillary overlap like roof tiles, called flap valves, permitting the influx of interstitial fluid. (See Fig. 4.) This process constitutes essentially the formation of lymph fluid.

Just as blood capillaries converge to form venules, then veins, lymphatic capillaries also unite to form increasingly larger tubes (again like the branches and twigs of a tree). Though these larger lymphatic vessels resemble veins structurally, they have thinner walls and more valves, which allow the lymph to move in one direction only.

Networks of lymphatic capillaries are distributed widely throughout the body. Yet some tissues lack lymphatic capillaries; these include avascular tissues (such as cartilage, the epidermis, the cornea of the eye), the central nervous system (the brain and spinal cord), splenic pulp, and bone marrow. In the small intestine, specialized lymphatic capillaries are called lacteals (*lact*, meaning "milky"). Located in the villi, they serve an important function in the absorption of fats and other nutrients, carrying dietary lipids (fats) into lymphatic vessels and ultimately into the blood. The presence of these lipids causes the lymph draining the small intestine to appear creamy white; such lymph is referred to as chyle ("juice"). In other areas, of course, lymph is a clear and pale fluid.

Comparison of the lymphatic vessels to the blood circulation is helpful in understanding some of the similarities between the two systems. Another similarity has to do with transport. The same factors that assist venous flow also affect lymph flow. These include breathing movements and muscle and joint "pumps"; in addition to aiding the return of venous blood back to the heart, they maintain lymph flow as well. The so-called respiration pump involves, of course, breathing in and breathing out (inhalation and exhalation). Pressure changes occur in this process, and this helps to move the lymph along. For example, when we take a deep breath (diaphragmatic breathing), lymph flows upward from the abdominal region, where the pressure is higher, toward the thoracic region, where it is lower. When we breathe out (exhalation), the pressure is reversed, yet the one-way valves in the vessels prevent the backflow of lymph. Through the contraction of smooth muscles in the walls of the lymphatic vessel, lymph is moved from one segment of the vessel to the next. Research has shown that thoracic duct lymph is literally "pumped" into the venous system during inspiration. The rate of flow is proportional to the depth of inspiration.

Also serving as lymph pumps are muscles and joints. When skeletal muscles, for example, contract, a "milking action" is created. This frequent intermittent pressure is put on the lymphatics to push the lymph forward. Most often this occurs during exercise and with general bodily movements. The contraction of muscles in both lymphatic vessels and veins force lymph eventually toward the subclavian veins (at the collarbones). Compared to the blood vascular system, however, the pressure moving through the vessels is very low. Squeezing the fluid along this one-way system will ultimately drain it into the venous system. So the flow of lymph from tissue spaces to the large lymphatic ducts to the subclavian veins is maintained primarily by the contraction of joints and skeletal muscles and by breathing movements. During exercise, however, lymph flow may increase as much as ten- to fifteen-fold.

Other pressure–generating factors that can compress the lymphatics also contribute to the effectiveness of the "lymphatic pump." These include arterial pulsations (pulse waves), postural changes, and passive compression of the body's soft tissues (manual lymph drainage therapy).

Even though there is no central pump, lymph vessels themselves assist in transporting and pushing lymph. They do this through a self-activated pumping motion found in the lymphangions, the section in the lymphatic vessel between two valves. The interaction between these valves and the musculature of the vessel wall makes the contractions that propel the lymph forward. Because of this function, these little angions are called "lymph hearts," which pulsate with an average frequency of ten per minute. In an X-ray, these vessels look like a string of pearls, with the string part representing the valves and the pearls the filled lymphangions. The ring–shaped muscles in the angions contain numerous nerve endings with connections to the autonomic nervous system; they are also influenced by the central nervous system. This is another way, along with the pumping motion, that the lymphangion functions like a "little heart." In conclusion, lymph drainage comes about as a result of the rhythmic, alternating dilations (expansion) and contractions of these "pearled" segments known as lymphangions.

CONCLUSION

After this rather technical introduction, a few concluding ideas to help summarize the concepts presented are needed here. Offering an overview of any bodily function that one can easily comprehend and grasp is difficult with any system, not only because of its overall complexity but because the understanding of the functioning of our body is a work in progress. Discoveries continue to be made, explorations continue to be done, revising former conceptions and rethinking old formulas.

The lymphatic system has several functions:

1. To drain interstitial fluid; this is the fluid that arises in between the cells; the lymphatic vessels help drain the tissue spaces from excess fluid

2. To transport dietary lipids (fats); these and other substances, such as proteins, are carried by lymphatic vessels and returned by them to the blood

3. To protect against invasion; lymphatic tissue carries out immune responses by targeting particular invaders or abnormal cells (such as bacteria, viruses, cancer cells, and so on) and responding to them in specific ways; in effect, destroying them and eliminating them from the body

Since blood and lymph are part of the circulatory system, comparisons between them may help in understanding more fully their role and function. Some differences include the following:

1. The lymphatic system does not form a complete and closed circuit like the blood.

2. The circulatory system has a muscular pumping organ—the heart; the lymphatic system does not.

3. Lymphatic capillaries structurally have larger diameters than blood capillaries and thinner walls than veins; also pressure is lower than in the blood vascular system.

4. The lymphatic network, unlike the blood, has "interruptions" by way of lymph nodes, stations which slow the movement of lymph temporarily in order to purify and filter the fluid.

Similarities between the two systems include the following:

1. Veins and lymphatic capillaries both have valves which move the fluid through the vessels; lymphatic vessels, however, have more valves.

2. Each forms increasingly larger structures, beginning with tiny capillaries and progressing to larger tubes and channels.

3. Respiration and joint/muscular movements affect transport for both.

4. Both are pervasive and widely distributed throughout the body.

These similarities and differences may assist in a better understanding of how the lymph operates in the physical body as well as the nature of its importance in our overall health and balance.

With the conclusion of this presentation, we will begin in the next chapter to study in greater detail the functioning of the lymphatic system as seen through the readings of Cayce. What were some of the indications, first of all, that pointed to improper lymph flow in the body?

How were these conditions described? What were the circumstances surrounding this dilemma? Recognition of the overall pervasiveness of the lymph will be one of the results from this examination.

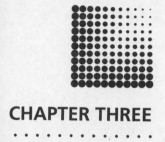

CHAPTER THREE

· · · · · · · · · · · · ·

Approaching a Balance:
Conditions Related to Lymph

In our desire and willingness to learn more about our physical body's wonderful activity, we discover that we also need to learn a new language to accompany the description of its functioning. We enter a fabulous world, ranging from microscopic particles invisible to the naked eye to masses of vital organs and tissues pulsating with energetic life. The processes and parts of our body require a fresh vocabulary to explain its workings, as we are approaching a whole new field of wonderment and exploration.

The health readings of Edgar Cayce add another dimension, another viewpoint, another level to our understanding and knowledge of our physical selves. They present, as stated in chapter 1, a holistic model of the body, interacting with and influenced by mind and spirit. This three–dimensional outlook, consistent throughout the readings, provides the dynamics upon which healing is based. When we take it upon ourselves to care for our bodies, no matter what health concern we are currently experiencing, we have a number of choices available to us to undertake this healing journey. Based upon a holistic concept, these choices include both allopathic and comple-

mentary therapies; thus, we can utilize the best combination of treatments from these two systems of medicine.

FURTHER REFLECTIONS ON CAYCE'S CONCEPTS

Through just a cursory examination of the Cayce physical readings
(which, by the way, are often difficult to comprehend even by medical
professionals), one gets a sense of what might be termed "the domino
effect"—that a certain result will follow a certain cause. If dominoes, for
example, are lined up in a row and the first one is tapped so that it falls,
the rest will fall, one after the other. During the Cold War era of Communism, this description was sometimes used to explain the potential
"fall" of certain nations to the effects of Communism's influence, perhaps being drawn in to this sphere by neighboring countries whose
governments had already collapsed to its evils. The Balkans, Southeast
Asia, and Central America are some examples of regions where the
spread of domination from one neighboring nation state to another
was feared, and the effort to forestall this from happening legitimized
U.S.-backed coups and other interventions. But the idea that one region
or country influences another and may indeed have a direct effect upon
another is reflected in our physical selves as well. This domino effect is
indicative also of the holistic nature of our bodies: one area being healed
or hurt affects another part.

Clients receiving massages at A.R.E.'s Health Center and Spa frequently report on feeling effects elsewhere in their body than where
the therapist's hands are working. While one client's head and neck
were being massaged, for example, she felt her toes tingle. Another client felt waves of energy going down his arms during his scalp massage.
Another woman whose shoulders were being rubbed felt heat in both
hips. Perhaps a release of energy took place that the body in its wisdom
distributed to areas where it was needed. Of course, this energy could
take the form of increased blood circulation, stimulation of nerve endings, relaxation of muscle tension, or simply an excess of healing energy from the therapist's hands that the body then carried to deficient
areas.

While this scenario of the domino effect probably occurs quite often as our physical bodies become more dis-eased over time, a number of play-by-play descriptions of this happening are offered in Cayce's readings. Though the terminology may be a bit unusual and the syntax convoluted, the message of the domino effect process, however, can still be understood. While lengthy, the following excerpt is a representative sample of such a scenario:

> In times back there were those reactions that have caused an unbalancing of the elements that go to make up what may be called a proper chemical balance necessary in the system. We had then an expression of what may be sometimes called a catarrhal condition, which developed in the sympathetic functioning system, by the amount of reduced circulation to the head, throat and nasal cavities. And this, tending to be of a drying nature, affected the muco-membranes especially in the upper portion, or in the head, antrum, nasal cavity, throat at times, the ears even. Not to the extent as to produce falling antrums or falling Eustachian tubes, yet these have been at times affected. This reducing then the quantity of the activity of the lymph circulation has caused lesions to form in various portions of the body, especially in the soft tissue; more adhesions than lesions, as related to muscular forces, though the toxic poisons that arise in the system from the poor eliminations (as it has affected throughout the system the lymph and emunctory circulation) cause the banking up of accumulations—or the lack of proper eliminations; affecting, to be sure, the blood supply, until we have an unbalanced condition in same, at times red blood running below normal and the white—especially in the leucocyte and the urea— making for lack of the quantity of blood in both its whole circulation and in its component parts. This is indicated by the character or type of distresses caused in same. For, at times we have had those experiences of a rash in the cuticle on various portions of the body. At other periods we have had occasionally a tendency for boils or abrasions, that cause considerable distress in portions of the system. At others we have found there were periods when the digestion was so upset as to find little that would assimilate properly with the body; tendency for keeping the body in rather a tautness. And lacking in replenishing powers made for these forms of adhesions in the antrum, the head, at times in the caecum—

as we have at the present, and an action that has tended to cause the
engorging of the colon; making for in the extremes, or in the lower
portions of the body, not exactly rheumatic conditions nor wholly
muscular reactions, but sciatic lumbago—these effects have been in the
system at various times.   642-1

According to the above excerpt, then, this forty–three–year–old
gentleman had earlier experienced a chemical imbalance that precipi-
tated "a catarrhal condition," an inflammation of the mucous membranes in the nose and throat areas. The eventual reduction in
circulation produced a drying effect in the head, throat, ears, antrum
(sinus cavity in the upper jaw), and nasal cavities. Lymph circulation
was also diminished, causing lesions in some soft tissues—adhesions
(fibrous tissue that abnormally joins body parts or tissues together) in
the muscles. A buildup of toxins or poisons caused by poor eliminations created the backing up of more accumulations, a condition which
affected the blood supply. Red blood and white blood supplies were at
times below normal. This circulation imbalance resulted in a number of
physical disturbances: a rash in the cuticles (outer layer of skin), boils,
abrasions, and periodic digestive upsets, so that he could not properly
assimilate his food. All of this kept him in a state of tension ("tautness"),
his body was thrown out of balance, and his colon became congested
(engorged), so that at various times he experienced what his reading
called "sciatic lumbago," or low pack pain.

The above reading was given on April 24, 1934, and Mr. [642] was
present for it. He had heard about Cayce's gift through an "automatic
writer," who had suggested that he study the A.R.E. group lessons, so he
organized a Search for God Study Group for that purpose.

Immediately following his reading he said that "the information fit-
ted his case perfectly and that there was no question in his mind as to
its correctness. He lamented the fact that so little credence was given
information of this kind, especially by the doctors." (642–1, R–1)

Later, in July 1934, he wrote:

About three months ago, Mr. Cayce gave me a physical reading. At that
time I was suffering from acute pleurisy, improper functioning of certain

glands of the head and throat, aggravated by adhesions in nasal cavities, and a general rundown condition, with a record of fifteen years of semi-invalidism.

The reading fully covered the conditions existent and gave treatment and diet, accompanied with manipulations by osteopathy.

Today I am enjoying nearly perfect health. I have endeavored to stay closely by [the] diet recommended, have taken the osteopathic treatments, and can say I cannot remember having enjoyed such health, as at present.

My case, I feel, is an unusual one, inasmuch as I have during the past fifteen years had three major operations, a severe accident with nine bones broken, three attacks of influenza, and typhoid fever, all of which has left me in an anemic, rundown condition. The remarkable phase of it all is that I feel 95 percent well in this brief period, having fully overcome constipation of long duration.

I gladly send this testimonial . . . I might add that three reputable medical diagnosticians and several practicing physicians have given me physical examinations prior to the reading by Mr. Cayce. Said examinations failed to reveal the causes of [my] disability, found in the reading.

Needless to say it is with much gratitude I express my appreciation to your organization, to Mr. Cayce, or I might say [to] the power which operates through Mr. Cayce.   642-1, R-3

Gladys Davis Turner, Cayce's longtime secretary, noted that the physical information contained in this letter was not known to Cayce consciously at the time of the reading. In August 1935 Mr. [642] obtained a check reading for his frequent headaches. In a follow-up letter, he wrote that he was very satisfied with this check reading, that it "meant more to me than to another, for it related to conditions and symptoms with which I labor." An additional notation in 1951 stated that he had remained active and interested in A.R.E. work.

Another satisfied customer, one might say. Following the advice given him in his reading paid off for him in better health and more vitality.

Similar to the domino effect, in which a lack or imbalance (the fall of a domino) in one area may precipitate a crisis or problem in another, the health readings oftentimes make reference to the importance of a cause–and–effect reaction. The cause, of course, would represent the seat of the problem, the main culprit, or perhaps the beginning point of the eventual disease process. It is most helpful to determine the cause or to pinpoint the initial stage of the illness, since addressing this area will often lead to a healing result more quickly and efficiently, as it is close to the origin of the imbalance.

Descriptions as to how this cause–and–effect scenario is played out may involve what sounds like battle or war terminology as the physical attempts to balance or aright itself after some type of attack or on-slaught. The infection–fighting cells—the white blood corpuscles, or leucocytes—are referred to as "warriors"; they attack the enemy, the in-vaders of the body, and their action alerts the body to the potential danger. How the physical responds is succinctly summarized in this statement from the readings:

> One should consider that the *system* is builded to *resist* whatever may arise, and it *takes that* direction in carrying out for what it *was* constructed, and when it meets obstructions; then it attempts to build around, or overcome, by *using* other portions or functionings to carry out its function.   943-17

It seems, then, that our physical bodies have a built–in mechanism that not only alerts the system to a potential danger but can even direct the influences needed to handle the situation, correct the imbalance, and relieve the "warlike" tension. The initial onslaught would be con-sidered "the cause" of the illness or ailment or distress. As for a reversal of the unhealthy condition, one reading states: " . . . the causes will not be relieved unless that which causes the conditions is relieved." (880–1)

Again, the importance of dealing with the cause is emphasized. The origin of a health concern can be a bit puzzling to uncover, much like locating the proverbial needle in a haystack. Many of Cayce's health readings pinpointed the cause; some informed the recipient of the read-ing that what was being addressed was an *effect* of imbalance, and *not* a cause. Often the seeker would simply ask for the cause of a particular ailment. One young man, twenty years old, asked: "What causes the eruptions on the skin, and can they be prevented by special diet or otherwise?" The answer came: "These are from poor eliminations and are a part of the system's attempt to adjust itself to changes that naturally come about." The reading suggested taking Eno Salts occasionally before breakfast, which would "assist in aiding the system to create a greater flow in the lymph and emunctory circulation . . . " (830-4) The circulatory system, the reading added, would eventually come into better balance.

Eno Salts is a laxative powder that was introduced in 1898 in Newcastle, London, as "Fruit Salt." Cayce seemed to prefer the fruit salts variety of eliminants. It was mentioned in more than 125 readings and also provides relief from indigestion, heartburn, upset stomach, and any discomfort after meals resulting from excess acidity.

The word *emunctory*, often mentioned in conjunction with lymph activity, refers to any organ or body part that gives off waste products, such as the skin, kidneys, or lungs. These are considered excretory organs, having to do with cleansing the body and ridding it of toxic substances.

For Mr. [830] the eruptions on his skin were caused from poor eliminations. For Mr. [829], who was suffering from cold, congestion, a tipped stomach, hernia, and noises in his ear, these conditions resulted from "disturbance in the circulation and the accumulations of an acidity in the system . . . [I]t is rather an effect and a result of disturbances than the nervous system being the cause of the conditions." (829-1) So for [829] the effect of his ailments was acidity and an imbalance in the circulatory system, the nervous system being the cause. The results of these disturbances brought a number of uncomfortable conditions. Suggestions for treatment included the use of an electric vibrator along the spine, wearing a support belt across the abdomen, applying hot salt and vinegar packs to his lower back, and adopting a largely alkaline diet. Although [829] was a participant in Study Group No. 11 of Washington, D.C., there is no follow-up or reports on his case.

Being aware of the domino effect and the cause–and–effect reaction in our body's attempts to maintain a homeostatic quality may help us in dealing with health concerns that we may be experiencing.

SOME INDICATIONS RELATED TO LYMPH FUNCTION

If the lymphatic system is doing its job properly—that is, the unhindered flow of fluid is transporting waste products, dead cells, proteins, and fats as well as vitamins and hormones back to the bloodstream—then our bodies would be in a balanced, well-defended state. "A healthy lymph system promotes healthy body tissues and body functions . . . It represents the omnipresent living environment of the body . . . " (Wittlinger, p. 14) But viruses and bacteria do exist, as they have for eons. Harmful substances, toxins, and injuries do provide external stimuli that may destabilize our system, causing damage, pain, and illness. So how do some of these effects manifest, especially in the health concerns and physical circumstances as presented to the sleeping Cayce?

Catarrh.   Probably the most obvious disturbances are those relating to catarrhal conditions. According to *The American Illustrated Medical Dictionary* by Dorland (1951), the word *catarrh* "has been practically eliminated from the scientific vocabulary" (p. 271); however, in its noun and adjective forms it appears quite regularly in Cayce's readings. Catarrh is an inflammation in the nasal and throat areas of the mucous membranes. These membranes line our body's inner cavities with a slick fluid so that substances can easily slip through and out of these inner tubes. Because of the preponderance of allergies or allergy-like symptoms, many people suffer from runny noses, itchy eyes, or sneezing fits as the body attempts to rid itself of the irritating allergen, the cause of the allergic reaction. For example:

> (Q) What is reason for excessive catarrhal discharge from head?
> (A) The system attempting to eliminate the excess conditions through
> the lymph circulation.   1266-4

Hydrotherapy treatments consisting of hot and cold baths plus massage were recommended to alleviate this condition for [1266].

Catarrhal conditions, however, while recognized primarily in the nasal passages, can also affect the entire system. Mucous membranes, as stated earlier, line interior body passages, so that a catarrhal condition can also exist in the stomach and intestines as well as in the head. One woman, so nervous she was taking sedatives, suffered from headaches, acidic stomach, and poor eliminations. Following a domino effect, her nervous condition produced "an irritation throughout the system," forming sacs in the abdominal area which disturbed the mucous membranes in the throat and head as well as the stomach and intestines, causing "a disturbance in the lymph circulation." (1288-1) She was advised to use the Wet-Cell Appliance, get osteopathic adjustments, take enemas, and follow a well-balanced diet, eating 80 percent alkaline-reacting foods. Unfortunately, no follow-up reports exist on her results.

In another reading, for a forty-one-year-old salesman who suffered from frequent headaches, this information regarding the pervasiveness of a catarrhal condition was submitted:

> There have been, as indicated, the effects upon the mucous membranes, upon the lymph circulation, from those infectious forces that arise from what is called a catarrhal condition—or the lymph and emunctory reaction that produces a force of infection in the system. It affects the body in much the same way as a rheumatic reaction, or a nervous reaction. For these conditions naturally in their very nature affect the nervous system, and especially in its relationships to muscular reaction . . .

As to its development and eventual effects, the reading added:

> . . . by exercise, by even small amount of draft that would be practically unnoticed by the body in its activities, by getting too warm in one way and manner or by cooling off too quickly, there is the reverberating—as it were—to the conditions that are existent. This makes for not only the repressions that produce headaches at times, hurt and burning of the eyes, but through cold or congestion a form of neuralgia that affects the head, the shoulders, and even the torso at times. All of these are but effects, as we find.   531-6

Because this was a follow-up check reading, slight corrections were made to his previous instructions, largely involving cleansing his system and increasing organ functioning. "Though requiring a little longer period, to eliminate the cause rather than the effects in the present will make for more permanent reaction in the body." (531-6) The man was advised to keep up the use of the Radio-Active Appliance (a device the readings stated several times was "good for everybody"), get a series of colonics ("to prevent or keep from causing a great deal of irritation from the infectious forces") and osteopathic adjustments ("that would make a stimulation to the *drainages* of the body"), and "Be mindful of the diets . . . " After some initial difficulty with the Radio-Active Appliance, he did follow the instructions and "was getting very good reactions with your treatment . . . while some days . . . I am not up to standard, I have come to realize that there is something good in what you are doing . . . " (531-6, R-6)

The next example is one probably many can relate to: "I have constant catarrh back of nose which runs down throat." (557-1) This fifty-two-year-old woman wondered if this condition were due to sinus trouble. The reading replied: "This is a natural condition from poor circulation in the lymph and emunctory activities of throat and head." In order "that the superficial circulation may be clarified by the cleansing and revivifying of the conditions," the Violet Ray hand machine was recommended as well as a nasal spray using water and Atomidine.

As a side note, the information in the Cayce health readings, as mentioned earlier, is very consistent in its holistic approach. In light of this quality Dr. Harold J. Reilly, a renowned physiotherapist who worked closely with a number of recipients of Cayce's readings, coined the acronym CARE and referred to the "Cayce CARE" therapy as a way of maintaining balance and health. The initials **C A R E** stand for **C**irculation, **A**ssimilation, **R**elaxation, and **E**limination, bodily processes that help to normalize the physical system and assist it in functioning more optimally. Some aspect of these four processes, implied either directly or indirectly, make up the bulk of the content of the health readings. Even in the short extracts or snippets from the readings included in this book, the reader needs to understand that the holistic concept of CARE is, nevertheless, included in the larger picture of health.

Sinusitis.   In the course of a year, an estimated thirty-seven million Americans experience sinusitis. It is the fifth most common diagnosis for which antibiotics are prescribed in outpatient settings. Sinusitis, an inflammation of the lining of the sinus cavities, is generally caused by an infection, allergies, irritants, or some obstruction. Four pairs of sinus cavities are connected by a passage to the nose. These cavities, which help to warm, moisten, and filter the air we breathe, are lined by membranes moistened by a thin mucus. Most cases of sinus infections are caused by viruses—so antibiotics would likely be ineffective.

In several instances in the readings, a sinus condition was attributed to "poor lymph circulation" (3187-1); another reading stated, "It is part of the lymph in the soft tissue . . . the slowing of the circulation makes for mucous accumulations in the sinus, see?" (2280-2) A sinus disorder was described in another reading as "the lymph flow through soft tissue" and resulted "from the slowed and disturbed circulation." (1023-1)

One woman asked this question: "What connection is there between either or both my hay fever and sinuses, with my asthma . . . ?" The answer was, "Well, all of these are associations with the lymph circulation, and with this engorgement these naturally cause—from the sinus—a general disturbance; as also does the hay fever." (3127-1)

What happens in the lymph system during an infection? It is as though a battle or a war were taking place within our bodies, which react to the invasion by assembling troops. The security forces are called upon. Our mucous membranes swell, while lymph vessels and nodes enlarge. The white blood cells destroy the invaders and remove them, taking them away like prisoners. However, if we have a poorly functioning lymph circulation, our defense system may be compromised. This circumstance, then, opens the door to an exacerbated condition, such as catarrh, sinusitis, chronic colds, sore throats, and so on. The resultant congestion, in other words, can be traced to a worsening and stagnation of lymph. (Chapter 6 will describe various methods to get the lymph circulation flowing more efficiently.)

Swelling.   Any abnormal enlargement of a body part is described as a swelling. When an abnormally large amount of fluid accumulates in connective tissue or intercellular spaces of the body or in body cavities, it is known as edema (also called dropsy). If the fluid accumulates in the tissue spaces and organs in the cavity of the abdomen, it is known as ascites.

A number of people occasionally experience puffiness in certain areas of their bodies, such as fingers, ankles, face, wrists, feet, or legs. For many, the condition is not serious, only symptomatic. While several causes exist for fluid retention, or swelling, by one's body, a few instances in the readings pointed to improper or poor lymph circulation. Here are some extracts as examples:

(Q) What is cause and cure for swelling on face?

(A) As indicated, there is the tendency for the emunctory [excretory] and lymph circulation to be so increased—by the humor created by subjugation in other portions of the body—as to create this activity.

Drainages set up by the stimulation of those centers as indicated, from the mechanical way and manner, will relieve these conditions.

275-41

This twenty-one-year-old woman harpist, who received this reading on May 17, 1934, was also experiencing erosion of the head of her femur (thighbone), which had first become apparent in February 1925. The recommendation of "Drainages . . . from the mechanical way and manner" referred to osteopathic adjustments, leading to successful relief of the swelling. In her later years, however, she wound up in a wheelchair, having to wear a brace, and eventually passed away on Thanksgiving morning, November 26, 1992, at the age of eighty.

On Halloween Day, October 31, 1930, a forty-year-old woman, according to the information in her reading (no background or follow-up reports and no check reading), had a hyperthyroid condition. She was also suffering from asthenia (weakness; loss of strength or energy), shortness of breath, poor circulation and digestion, and pleurisy. The reading noted the swelling in her limbs, ankles, and feet and the cause: "This is the lack of *lymph* circulation, or may be termed oppositely, in that the *lymph* is *full* without the *proper* amount of pressure *in* the lower extremities to carry circulation *back* properly." (130-1)

The reading advised the Wet-Cell Appliance with iodine solution gradually added to create a proper balance in her digestive system; osteopathic manipulations; a diet rich in iron, calcium, silicon, and phosphorus; plenty of rest; a moderate amount of exercise; and mullein stupes for the "swollen side, caused by pleurisy and swollen veins."

When she asked how long it would take "to bring the body to normal," this answer, reflecting the balance between mind and body, was given:

> In three to five weeks, as given, there will be the *definite* change for the betterment of the body. As to the responses from then on, will depend upon the conditions in the body itself—the mental attitude, the rate of vibration as is kept, and the activities of same. Don't eat too much—don't get scared—don't work too fast—don't think too hard!   130-1

Imbalances in pressure, mentioned a number of times in the readings, are responsible in part for poor lymph flow, as in [130]'s case above. For Mrs. [1433], who received her first of ten readings on August 27, 1937, and was suffering from uricacidemia (an accumulation of uric acid in the blood), this comment was offered:

> *In the nervous system,* we find the pressures from poisons that dilate the emunctory and the lymph centers produce a little swelling in the lower limbs and the knees, about the abdomen, and those areas in the brachial centers and the limbs in the upper portion of the body—all cause acute conditions from pressures and from the poisons in the system.   1433-1

A series of sal soda (washing soda) packs was recommended as well as Toris Compound (a laxative preparation), colonics, adjustments, the Wet-Cell Appliance with atomic iodine (Atomidine), and a diet of more vegetables, fewer starches. She had difficulty in getting help to follow her readings, required nursing care, and in 1942 a routine mailing to her address was returned unclaimed.

One fifty-five-year-old man asked in his reading about a small swelling on the left side of his spine. It was neither red, inflamed, nor painful, so it did not really bother him.

> This is an accumulation of lymph. The Glyco-Thymoline Packs should be applied over this area, for these will take away the pressures that have been causing other disturbances in the body. Let the Packs be applied about twice a week, leaving them on until the two or three thicknesses

of cotton cloth have dried out from the body absorption.   3079-2

In his next reading, he was advised to continue the packs, "for through this means [the packs] we are gradually reducing the tendency for the accumulation of lymph pockets in the tissue through those areas." (3079-3) The term *lymph pockets* was used in a number of readings, suggesting the formation of sacs or pouches where excessive lymph accumulates. These pockets, if not dissipated over time, seem to be the forerunner of cysts, hence the encouragement in [3079]'s reading to continue use of the Glyco packs to prevent cyst formation.

Another reading made a reference to the possibility of the formation of tumors, as a condition of a swollen abdomen. This forty–five–year–old woman apparently was diabetic, according to the information in her reading ("too great a quantity of sugars for a nominal balance"), and overweight. In her only reading (no background information or follow-up reports), she asked just two questions: about the pain in her back and the swelling in her abdomen. She wondered if she had a tumor. The response to her latter question was that the swelling was a "natural reflex . . . It is only of the lymph and emunctory circulation, which *causes* puffing or fullness, but not in any form tumorous in its nature—as yet." (2338-1) A series of osteopathic manipulations to stimulate eliminations (which would also alleviate her back pain) was recommended as well as a series of wet heat applications to the lower end of her spine. Her diet should include Jerusalem artichokes (for assimilation), no fried foods or red meat, and plenty of vegetables. "Do these things as indicated; we will not only remove the disturbances but *prevent* a great deal of disturbance later . . . " (2338-1)

One final reading in this section on swelling also mentions a "reflex" action as well as the close connection of the lymphatic with the blood circulation. A woman psychologist (no age given) received a reading on July 7, 1923; her two sisters and her husband also obtained readings. She asked the cause of the swelling in her legs, and this was the response:

The circulation is as we have given here, lymphatic forces separating themselves between the arterial or venous circulation. When it gets to portions of the body, then with the body standing, this produces the inability of the condition to be brought back to eliminate . . . This is reflex, one from the other, you see. Give the forces to the system as we have outlined, and we will overcome this condition, you see, permanently. 4889-1

The "forces to the system" outlined in her reading included a diet rich in iron plus plenty of fruits (berries that grow close to or on the ground), pears, and "some kind of peaches, though not all." A special tonic formula was advised plus exercise. In addition, she was told: "Keep the mind forces well in attune with the developing physical force and lift up the body to this element. Do that." (4889-1) No follow-up medical reports or subsequent readings are on file.

CONCLUSION

In our physical body's efforts to combat imbalances, which may have been spurred by a domino effect, we can take a certain amount of comfort from the positive suggestions found in the Cayce readings: the potential for cure or relief of the distress is readily available provided the recommendation is followed, the advice is carried out, the remedies are applied. The scope of this book, however, while offering in condensed form a list of certain treatments and suggestions from individuals' readings, is not intended as a how-to text, but to present a broad overview of the function of the lymph, as reiterated in the Cayce health information. More than three thousand references to the words *lymph, lymphatic,* or *lymphatics* occur in the readings (in slightly over two thousand documents), totaling about one-third of the entire body of health readings. While this chapter covered briefly just three conditions relating to the lymph—catarrh, sinusitis, and swelling—the next chapter will explore additional indications from the readings in which the lymphatic system was directly or indirectly involved.

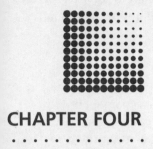

CHAPTER FOUR

Additional Conditions Related to Lymph

It is a natural inclination within us: when we become ill or notice some type of irregularity in our bodies, we want to correct it, to make it right, to return to our normal, usual healthy state. Those recipients of Cayce's health readings were no different. Having access to this remarkable source of what many consider today accurate information, they were the lucky ones who had the opportunity to avail themselves of such insight and knowledge. Because of Cayce's selfless service and loving concern for others, we are the beneficiaries of his more than fourteen thousand readings, two-thirds of which deal with health concerns. Now with fairly easy access to this wealth of information, we can research, study, and contemplate these treasures and try for ourselves the suggested treatments. **(Note: Any of the recommended suggestions for treatment should be used under the supervision of a health professional.)**

With few exceptions, all of the physical readings were given for individuals with different needs, hence the slight variations that may appear from one reading to another, especially in those with similar conditións (for example, differences in dosage, manner of application, or formula). Yet within this body of information, as stated earlier, lies a principle of whole-ness—with its physical, mental, and spiritual aspects—that can be universally applicable to all. In this spirit is presented here those excerpts to help the reader comprehend more fully the workings of the human body with regard to the lymphatics.

COOPERATIVE SYSTEM

Each bodily system performs as though it were a separate entity in carrying out its particular function. One of the difficulties, however, in discussing a single body system in isolation is the fact that these systems don't function entirely alone; they are interdependent, affecting each other in a truly operating spirit of cooperation, so that it is impossible to talk about one without involving another. Take digestion as an example. The food we eat naturally goes through a transformative process to become converted to the energy we need to maintain life; however, if we engage our muscular system to a great extent by working out at a gym following a heavy meal, we risk the ill effects of nausea or cramping because the digestive process has been interrupted. In another instance, as important as oxygen is to our blood supply, for inhalation and exhalation we need our muscular system and bone structure to enable our lungs to work smoothly and correctly. The lymphatic structure as well overlaps or affects other systems, helping and supporting those systems to easily carry out their work, or it can—in the case of dis-ease—compromise or inhibit their function. As part of the immune system, the lymph assists in defending our body against invading organisms that may cause infection or disease, but if we are not eliminating regularly and efficiently through the proper channels, toxins build up in us and we become ill.

Lymph, like blood, flows through a very extensive network of tubes; in a sense, it is everywhere, transporting particular substances and returning them to the general circulation. It also cycles through the excretory organs—called in the readings "emunctories"—where various wastes are discarded. A number of times the Cayce readings make reference to the lymph and the emunctories as if they were one unit; the readings also frequently mention the influence of the lymph on the digestive system, the nervous system, and the circulatory system. What are some of the results, then, of the lymph's impact on these bodily systems as experienced by those who had received readings from Cayce? For what particular problems or discomforts did they seek solutions? Starting at the external, let's examine skin conditions as related to the lymphatic system.

THE SKIN: OUR LARGEST ORGAN

The importance of our skin is ably demonstrated by Frederick Rossiter's quote in *Water for Health and Healing:*

> The skin on a human being is the largest, heaviest organ of the body. It takes about 17 square feet of skin to cover the average man or woman . . . the entire skin is one great sentient membrane of closely knit nervous and vascular tissues . . . It has been estimated that in one square inch of true skin there are several millions of cells of various tissues, several feet of minute blood tubes, a dozen feet of nerve fibres, one hundred sweat glands and a score of oil glands. p. 34

So the skin isn't merely a protective wrapping in which we're encased; it's an organ system with various specific functions: it regulates body temperature, senses both painful and pleasant stimuli, prevents substances from entering the body, and shields us from the sun's harmful rays. Our individuality is also marked by the texture, folds, and colors of our skin, so that if something interferes with our skin's function or appearance, it can have consequences on our physical and mental health.

Here are some skin conditions in which the Cayce information made a reference to their connection with the lymphatic system:

Psoriasis. A chronic disease that affects the skin, causing bright red lesions covered by thick, dry, silvery scales, bumps, or various-sized patches on the skin, psoriasis appears in 2–4 percent of white people (blacks are less likely to get it). While a number of causes and treatments are outlined in the readings, one comment stands out starkly:

(Q) Is psoriasis always from the same cause?
(A) No, but it is more often from the lack of proper coordination in the eliminating systems. At times the pressures may be in those areas disturbing the equilibrium between the heart and liver, or between heart and lungs. But it is always caused by a condition of lack of lymph circulation through [the] alimentary canal and by absorption of such activities through the body.   5016-1

The alimentary canal, also known as the gastrointestinal (GI) tract, is a continuous, hollow, muscular tube that coils and winds through the body cavity, beginning at the mouth and ending at the anus, the outlet of the rectum. It comprises the main organs of the digestive system: the mouth, pharynx, esophagus, stomach, and small and large intestines. According to this reading excerpt, then, improper or deficient lymph circulation throughout this tract and its consequent poor "absorption of such activities through the body" (nondelivery of the proper nutrients extracted from the digestion process) lead to a psoriatic condition in the body.

A thirty-five-year-old floral decorator received a reading on June 7, 1943, which seems to reconfirm the lymph and psoriasis connection. She had read a review of *There Is a River* (the Cayce biography by Thomas Sugrue) in the *Sunday Times* and "felt immediately with more joy that I can express that the answer to my problem of years' standing was solved . . . I have since read the book and feel only more firmly convinced . . . " (3032-1, B-1) She had suffered from psoriasis for twenty-two years, since she was thirteen, and had gone to numerous doctors and skin specialists, "but no cure for it is known to the medical world . . . " She further described her condition:

These unsightly red blotches practically cover my arms and legs, and part of the abdomen and have been a great source of discomfort and embarrassment. Recently it has spread to my hands.

For some time I have felt that psoriasis is, in some way, connected with the mind, and perhaps a karmic result. Being a person who has had numerous complexes and mental problems, much of which I have been able to overcome through study in metaphysics, I still feel I am not wholly adjusted at this point . . .   3032-1, B-1

She requested also a life reading to assist her "toward a more complete mental adjustment and spiritual growth . . . " In fact, both the physical and life reading were taken on the same day. Her physical reading picked up immediately on her psoriatic condition, noting a "thinning of the walls in the intestinal system. Thus the activities of the lymph and emunctory circulations through these portions carry that humor into the lymph circulation, which causes that irritation to the skin called psoriasis." (3032-1) A series of colonics followed by needle showers and a massage was suggested along with dietary advice. She was pleased with the reading, went to see Dr. Harold Reilly for the treatments, and promised to "follow the reading closely and write you the results. I am so thrilled at the prospect of having clear healthy skin and already I feel less fatigued and considerably more ease of body." (3032-1, R-2) She also derived great benefit and inspiration from her life reading, which gave her "direction and polarization of which I was badly in need." Unfortunately, no follow-up information exists.

Another person was experiencing a skin condition with "eruptive forces, scaly places, or swellings" as well as abrasions on different parts of her body, particularly on the scalp. These conditions, the reading explained, were due to "the lymphatic circulation attempting to take from the blood supply and to carry out through the pores of the skin those poisons as are *not* being eliminated through the activities of the excretory forces in the liver proper." Diet and osteopathic adjustments were some of the recommendations for alleviating this incoordination and would assist "the system in ridding from the body those poisons that are *still* carried in the lymphatic circulation, that *should* be eliminated through the alimentary canal." (337-4) An overloaded or overtaxed eliminating system was a common culprit in many unhealthy conditions, in this case causing scaly outbreaks on the skin.

Boils.   A similar situation to psoriasis-like conditions is the outbreak of boils: tender, swollen areas caused by staphylococcal infection around hair follicles. The pus-filled nodules are frequently found on the neck and buttocks but can develop on any area where a break in the skin allows bacteria to penetrate the skin's outer layer. Consider another cause presented in this question–and–answer extract:

> (Q) What is cause and remedy for boils on back of neck?
>
> (A) The eliminations . . . should so clarify and purify the blood as to make for better eliminations; and the incoordination in eliminations . . . is that which produces this tendency for poisons to be eliminated by eruptions in the lymph circulation.   389-5

Again, an imbalance or lack of coordination in the eliminating system resulted in these skin eruptions.

In a previous reading, this person was told that a "regurgitation through the stomach" was the natural result of "not taking sufficient rest before activities after meals, or from an *unbalanced* meal with too much greases that are not easily assimilated . . . " (389-4) An interesting comment added by the reading was that lymph circulation through portions of the intestinal tract had been reduced as a result—similar to the cause of psoriasis cited earlier in reading 5016-1.

Pimples. Long the bane of teenagers, pimples are an unsightly skin disturbance that, depending upon its origin, can affect all ages. One twenty–year–old woman, who had pimples even on her scalp, asked why her skin was so irritated. The response was familiar: "The poor eliminations or the disturbances between the eliminating channels of the body, because of this disturbance in the lymph circulation throughout the body." (3465-1) However, she was also told that owing to a previous injury to the wall of her vagina, she had a tendency toward "a hooded womb," and the stress on her nervous system just before her menstrual periods exacerbated her condition. Adjustments to correct the position of the pelvic organs were recommended. Yet, according to the information in her reading, this condition had created throughout her body a disturbance in her lymph circulation.

Erysipelas. An acute infectious disease of the skin or mucous membranes, erysipelas is caused by streptococcus. It is usually characterized by round or oval patches on the skin which enlarge and spread, becoming red, swollen, and tender, sometimes accompanied by small blisters. It is a form of cellulitis. One reading referred to this disease as "a lymph disturbance" (1014-1); however, this forty–one–year–old man had other physical conditions that were causing a drain upon his sympathetic nervous system and blood supply. Three other cases in the readings, the subjects ranging in age from thirteen months to twenty-four years, refer to erysipelas (plus one with a tendency to the disease), yet other complications were mainly addressed with no specific reference to lymph.

Dry skin. While dry skin can conceivably have many causes, in a number of instances in the readings, the condition was traced to lymph. Described as a causal factor in one reading as "lack of the lymph through the superficial circulation" (5391-1), another mentioned "the very poor lymph circulation at times, causing a dryness or dullness to the superficial circulation . . . " (3175-2) Another's "dryness to the skin, over portions of the body [was] from the attempt of the lymph to supply the necessary influences for drainages . . . " (1771-1) Again, these are instances of impedance of lymph circulation.

Eczema. Also called dermatitis, eczema is an inflammation of the skin's upper layers, resulting in blisters, redness, itching, scaling, and swelling. One reading described its origin as "congestions in the lymph circulatory forces", implying some kind of blockage, or lack of flow, that creates a buildup of wastes in the eliminating channels. (1383-1)

A twenty-nine-year-old woman with dermatitis had a second reading from Cayce, in which she asked:

(Q) Why is it that when I get tired itching usually results?
(A) This is the effect of the lack of flow of lymph from the nerve exhaustion to the superficial portion of the circulation. These are those supplies needed, as indicated by the type of adjustments and treatments, as well as the type of tonic as we would take.   2551-2

According to a notation made following her first reading,

Her skin gets extremely dry and caky all over the body, not a place that is not affected. The itching is torment—she scratches off the scales, and then applies oil—to keep the skin lubricated and to prevent the constant toughening. Years ago her skin was like an elephant's, though this time it doesn't get as bad as that—but she suffers just as much; has said that

she would kill herself, if she had the courage, when she feels one of the
itching attacks coming on.   2551-1, R-1

Unfortunately, no follow-up reports exist. According to her reading,
the initial problem was the result of a glandular imbalance, creating
both pathological and psychological disturbances. The tonic referred to
was beef juice; she was also to receive massages with peanut oil, treatments with the Mercury Quartz Light, positive suggestions, and osteopathic adjustments.

Blemishes.   Because of an extremely disturbed condition in the blood
supply, according to reading 1012-1, "the coordination between the
lymph and the deeper circulation and the superficial" was impaired,
which made for "blemishes on parts of the body." The reading indicated
that it was specifically referring to an area on the body's left side that
had earlier been bruised "from a lick or from striking against the corner
of something." A skin tumor arose as a result. Frequently the readings
noted such tumors originating because of undue pressure, blows, or
repetitive injuries to the same area. After being given a particular formula, this woman was told to gently massage around and over the area
of the lump. No specific follow-up reports on her health exist, but in
1961 Gladys Davis noted that she was still apparently in good health
and active in her job. She visited the A.R.E. headquarters in Virginia
Beach in 1981.

Bones: Our Support System

When one considers the skeletal system, one thinks of the bony, hard
material that gives shape and strength to our bodies and helps form
our physical appearance. In addition to providing this support structure, our bones also help protect vital, delicate, internal organs, such as
the brain and heart, and manufacture blood cells and platelets in the
marrow. They serve as areas of attachment for muscles and enable us
through the joints to move, sway, bend, and turn in numerous directions.

A number of people who had readings complained of bone or joint
problems and requested help in dealing with them. Here are a few of
those situations:

Arthritis.   Inflammation of a joint is called arthritis. A potentially de-bilitating and crippling disease, it was described in one reading as a "stiffening or crystallizing, as it were, of the tendon and muscular forces." (631–6) This thirty–seven–year–old woman had asked about the swelling in her knees, ankles, and left hand, and the reading stated it was "the effect of the arthritic activity in the system, or too great a quantity of the salts of the system . . . Or the lack of sufficient quantity of lymph circulation." Then, the reading continued with a fuller expla-nation:

> For arthritis is, in its incipiency or in its greater activity, an attack upon the lymph circulation; either by the lack of activities in the secreting glands of the system to supply sufficient oils and nutriment for the muscular and tendon forces, that is experienced first in extremities as in hands, knees, feet or elbows or the like, or all combined. First it is a disturbance in the circulation, really a disturbance in the lymph circulation, and is a portion of this distress in this body of [631] in the present.   631-6

Thirteen different categories exist for arthritis, according to the Ar-thritis Foundation and the American Rheumatic Association, and the causes range from infection and the normal aging process and genetics to physical or emotional stress or simply unknown factors. For the indi-vidual in the above reading, the lack of lymph circulation also resulted in fewer nutrients and lubricating oils being supplied to the muscles and tendons; this would indicate perhaps a rheumatoid condition which involves changes in connective tissues (muscles, tendons, bursae, and fibrous tissue) as well.

Cracking/creaking joints.   Joints are formed where the ends of bones come together. They generally provide motion and flexibility, except in areas where they are fused. Probably most of us have experi-enced the creaking, cracking, or popping noises that seem to emanate from the joints, such as when we crack the knuckles in our fingers or toes. Most of these sounds, however, are probably due to a tight muscle or ligament rolling and snapping over the joint as it is being moved. In fact, this was so stated in the following:

(Q) What causes creaking bones in upper region of shoulders and spine, and what corrective measures are necessary?
(A) The stimulation for a more uniform activity of the circulation as related to the lymph and emunctory activity through the portions should supply the necessary burses about the joints and bones for this to be entirely eliminated. The tendency arises from too little a circulation of the lymph and emunctory, especially about the tendons and muscles. It isn't the bones that creak; it's the muscular contraction.   270-32

Here are a few other questions in the readings regarding the cause of this noise:

(Q) What is cause of creaking joints?
(A) Lack of proper circulation, or—as might be termed—it needs oiling up; that is, more of a lymph circulation. Hence those vital energies as given, of the vital forces to act with body functioning.   1688-9

(Q) What is causing the cracking in joints?
(A) The lack of the fluids in those areas. Lack of lymph.   849-40

It makes sense, then, that for the joints to work more smoothly and with less noise, additional lubrication would be needed.

One twenty–year–old woman asked what could be done to stop her jaw from cracking. This reply was given:

This is a condition that is produced by the activity of the lymph circulation, and under the existent conditions is the outcome of that being attempted to be produced in the system. It is a natural consequence. It is not of such a nature to be objectionable, though it becomes at times to the body rather troublesome. But as conditions are balanced, this will gradually disappear.   275-31

Knots. Although knots or hard lumps may be associated with arthritis as the bony tissue becomes more calcified, in the following case this thirty–year–old man had problems with a stiff finger (doctors told him the finger was dead) plus knots that would appear and disappear on his fingers, feet, and face. Here is a portion of his reading's explanation:

> This is the incoordination . . . that arises from the lymph circulation. It is
> bettered, as we find—that is, the circulation. In overtaxing of the body,
> this is when these accumulations or knots appear. Then when there is
> the perfect relaxation, these disappear.   533-18

He was advised to take Adiron to "keep better and stronger activity throughout the body." (Originally known as Codiron, Adiron contained cod liver oil and was a source of vitamins A, B, D, E, and G.) The reading continued with two more recommendations:

> Also the disturbances will be less and less by the use of the massages
> of the Peanut Oil externally, as well as the Olive Oil internally. Use the
> Peanut Oil massage for the feet and limbs, body, face and neck, at least
> once a week. This, absorbed, will also aid in keeping the conditions
> thinned in the epidermis circulation, so that these accumulations will not
> be caused.   533-18

Three-and-a-half months later, following a check reading, he reported that the information did him "a world of good," and four years later, in reply to a questionnaire, he stated, "I am able to take any activity desired now." (533-19, R-4)

A fifty-one-year-old woman with a variety of complaints received thirty-nine readings. In her eleventh one she asked a question about the enlarged joints in her hands. The reading explained:

> Most of it is hard work and worry, and acid in system! The *lymph
> producing* those—hence the vibrations to carry these *away from* the
> central portion and distribute them to their *normal* eliminations, see?
>   243-11

Relating an acidic condition of the blood to joint disturbances was a frequently stated correlation in the Cayce readings. In this woman's case hard work plus worry added to the condition, perhaps indirectly contributing to and exacerbating her body's acidity. The treatments or remedies ("vibrations") to help alleviate the problem, "to carry these *away from* the central portion [of the body] and distribute them to their *normal* eliminations" would consist of, according to a statement earlier in her reading, Citrocarbonate, Milk of Magnesia, and Milk of Bismuth. ("These . . . will tone the stomach.") Not only were her joints enlarged, they were also giving her a burning sensation, which occurred as well "in the fleshy part of body." This also was due to too much acid, the reading said, then added: "Hence those absorptions as are given in that of the Milk of Bismuth, with those of Citrocarbonates that will act upon the *lymphs* of the system and the emunctory circulation; while those properties of the Magnesia will make for better eliminations." (243–11) She continued to experience health challenges, eventually dying in 1957 in her seventies.

Joint pain. This, of course, is a very common complaint that seems to affect most of us at one time or another, even if for brief periods. A forty–one–year–old music teacher asked in his reading what was caus- ing the pain in his joints. The answer came: "As indicated, the lack of the lymph flow and the lack of the eliminations to keep away the poisons produced by the excess of temperature through the circulatory forces of the body." (1476–2) The reading was given on December 31, 1937. In April 1951 Hugh Lynn Cayce, Edgar's son, met Mr. [1476] in Los Angeles. He had begun losing the use of his hands and was unable to continue working as a pianist. He mentioned that he wished he had followed his reading, which predicted the worsening condition unless the cause was removed. Diet, massage along the cerebrospinal system with "*high* vi- brations of electrical forces," colonics, and occasional fume baths had been recommended.

A fifty–two–year–old woman wondered what was causing the sore- ness in her left knee. The reading indicated that it was from "a tendency towards neuritis, which—of course—is nerve pressure or soreness, from the lack of lymph flow to those portions." (2025–1) As in a number of physical readings, a hopeful note was added: "This will disappear en- tirely as the other corrections are made as indicated." (2025–1) Unfortu- nately, the follow-up information made no mention of her sore left knee.

Neuritis is an inflammation of a nerve that attacks the peripheral nerves, the nerves that link the brain and spinal cord with the muscles, skin, organs, and all other parts of the body. Because these nerves usually carry sensory and motor fibers, the result can be both painful and paralytic. Bell's palsy, sciatica, and tic douloureux are special types of neuritis; neuralgia is a form of neuritis in which pain is the chief symptom. According to this reading, the lack of lymph flow resulted in this neuritic tendency.

SENSORY ORGANS

Our five senses deliver to us information and cues about our external world, and to a great extent, we have learned to function and operate based upon their data. The physiological functions of these organs—sight, taste, smell, hearing, and touch—provide a central sensory input from highly specialized receptor cells located in our eyes, mouth, nose, ears, and skin. When our senses detect something, they register its presence through the nerve signal, which goes along sensory nerves to the brain. Our nervous system helps us interpret what is continually being presented to us. Yet these sensory inputs overlap, and what we eventually experience is actually a blending of stimulus effects.

The term *sensory organs* appears in more than eighty readings, while the term *sensory forces* occurs over 450 times. In many of these instances, a wider and broader meaning of the senses is intended. Consider the following selected extracts:

Eyes.   One man asked the cause of his blurred eyesight. Earlier in the same reading, he had been told that an infection in his blood produced "an inflammatory condition affecting the nerves, the muscular forces, the tendons in other portions of the system," causing "a strain upon the lymph circulation." A blood test taken earlier showed that he had a syphilitic infection, and this check reading confirmed it. The "same pressure in the lymph circulation" was affecting his eyesight. The reading explained further that the "strain by the use of the eyes carries the inflammation to the mucous membranes or around the ball and makes, as it were, a fogginess more than a dimness." (862-2) He was to continue his treatments, especially occasional massages to the upper dorsal (thoracic) and cervical (neck) areas.

A subsequent letter from his great-niece indicated improvement in

his eyes through use of the Wet–Cell Appliance and sticking to the recommended diet. Later, however, he discontinued use of the appliance
"because his wife cannot understand the purpose for same and here
again he must meet his own results." (862–6, R–1)

A forty–one–year–old salesman, whom we met in chapter 3 under
the heading "Catarrh," wondered if he needed glasses because, as he
stated, "I seem to get a glare—affecting eyesight, etc." The reading pointed
to the cause: "Such effects are from pressures that are hindrances, especially through the lymph circulation, through soft tissue in face, head
and neck, by congestion and accumulations of poisons." (531–6) He
would only need glasses, the reading noted, if he didn't follow the suggestions indicated. Though he had difficulty following some of the recommendations—the appliance and colonics—he stated three months
after the reading, "I have been feeling fair, but will try to live more in
the regime set, only I haven't the time right along." (531–6, R–4)

Mouth.   In one particular case, a seventy–eight–year–old woman
asked, "What causes my mouth to get dry?" (1477–1) She was also bothered by an ear infection, a stiff neck, and hypotension. The reading
explained that "the circulations are not coordinating," and this produced
variations in temperature in her hands and feet as well as in other
portions of her body. This deflected circulation is what was causing the
dry condition in her mouth, affecting her salivary glands. In a domino
effect the drying up of the salivary glands caused "lack of nourishment
or lymph flow there." Unifying these "would release the energies in such
a manner as to bring the renewed forces to the system." She was advised
to use the Radio–Active Appliance, which "would produce the coordination of the deep circulation, the superficial circulation, and a stimulation to the activity of the glandular system." No follow–up reports are
on file.

On May 31, 1944, a sixty–seven–year–old artist and art instructor received his only reading. He wrote a few weeks earlier that he had been
helped a great deal spiritually ("more than I can say") by the biography
of Cayce, *There Is a River* by Thomas Sugrue. He had several health concerns: floaters in his eyes, pains in his stomach and abdomen ("I suspect
that I have taken poison in food"), fatigue, and ringing in ears (5183–1,
B–2). The reading mentioned some of these conditions in addition to a

prostate problem and recommended fume baths, massages, short-wave treatments, and colonics. Included in his reading was also this question-and-answer exchange:

> (Q) What can be done to prevent dribbling, which occurs now and then?
> (A) This is a part of too much stimulation from the cervical, and as these areas are brought more in accord there will be better circulation and lack of too much lymph through the salivary glands, and the general conditions will be better through other portions of head, shoulder and neck.
>
> 5183-1

After a few months' delay, he received his hydrotherapy treatments at the Reilly Health Service in Rockefeller Center in New York City but experienced no definite improvement in his condition. He reported frequency of urination (from prostate problems), breathing difficulties, and poor eyesight—all of which his reading traced to toxemia. Yet he remained enthusiastic about the Cayce information and, following Cayce's death in January 1945, wished to help continue the work. In reply to a 1949 questionnaire, he noted: "Much improved, although mild recurrences do happen. I am not continuing the treatments as recommended in my first physical reading." (5183-1, R-3)

On January 15, 1936, a longtime A.R.E. supporter (who eventually became a Life member) received his twentieth reading, requested because of a severe cold and congestion. Previously, he had gotten help for a longstanding condition of gastritis.

> (Q) Do you note anything in roof of mouth and around tongue?
> (A) Only the fullness as produced by excess of the lymph circulation, and accumulations in the area. The hot applications to the feet and to the lumbar and sacral area will pull the blood away from these.
>   And the enemas to make for the assimilations to become eliminations for the necessary forces of the body.
>
> 261-20

Two weeks after receiving the reading, he wrote, "I have had quite a siege here, but finally seem to be on the upgrade." (261-20, R-1) In general, he appeared to follow the suggestions in his readings with good success. His wife and daughter also received readings. After receiving his final reading, he wrote: "For some time after receiving the reading I felt considerably better. If I don't now it is only because I don't continue to do all the things the reading recommended. I am so very busy these days that I find it hard to do all the things that I should." (261–35, R–1) A familiar situation!

Nose. Toxemia is a condition in which bacterial products or poisonous substances (toxins) are spread throughout the body via the bloodstream. The term is frequently used in the readings as a description of one's physical health, usually resulting in a myriad of problems—from swelling and pain to high blood pressure and various incoordinations. These were some of the symptoms experienced by one woman, who asked, "What causes the feeling of a cold coming on in nose and head, but never developed?" The answer given also included the remedy:

> Lack of proper eliminations through the lymph circulation. Hence as indicated the treatments for the perspiratory system, or mild sweats; not being too heavy on heart, but these are necessary to set up better stimulation through the whole system.   494-6

Her son had requested this reading, her final one; in her previous readings, no age is given. The caution in the excerpt about the effect of sweat baths on the heart was given because she had been experiencing fluctuations in her blood pressure. Despite an operation to correct a prolapsed uterus, she had been improving, but no further details are given following this last reading.

Ears. In this twelfth reading for [4281], a seven–year–old girl suffering from the aftereffects of malaria, an increase in lymphatic circulation was putting "distress through the bronchials, nasal cavities, and through that of the thyroids and the portions of the throat proper . . . " The reading went on to state that "[a]ll the portions of the throat, and all the conditions in the lymphatic circulation, as we see, are involved . . . " (4281–12) The Eustachian tube was also affected, and this was the cause of her earaches. Because her system became "easily excited or exaggerated by an increased circulation," she was advised to massage coco-quinine (cocoa butter and quinine) in the lymph areas: arm pits, elbows, abdomen, and thighs. This would reduce capillary circulation, allowing the lymphatics to take it up. Some exercise, but not getting overheated, was also recommended.

A little over two weeks later, a letter stated that she was showing improvement, "though slowly." (4281-12, R-1) She was still running a temperature and had spent some time in a sanitarium in Decatur, Georgia, where she had made moderate improvement. She received her final reading at nine years of age in which Cayce said, "The body is in very good condition . . . Developing, both mentally and physically—and very good." (4281-17)

A fifty-one-year-old woman wrote to Edgar Cayce on June 21, 1943. She had just read *There Is a River* and was impressed with Cayce's clairvoyant ability to diagnose illnesses and prescribe treatments. A practical nurse who loved her work, she nevertheless was troubled by a variety of ailments, many stemming from an injection with a hypodermic needle that had penetrated the bone covering, depositing its contents there instead of in the bloodstream. This resulted in intestinal adhesions and arthritis of the spine. She also had a calcified lump in her chest, receding gums, and lack of endurance. On November 3, 1943, she obtained her reading, which began: "Has been a very lovely person!" (3334-1) The reading addressed her complaints and answered her question about a ringing in her ears: " . . . this is the lack of the lymph circulation, caused by congestion of the emunctory patches through portions of the body centers." In general, her body's various incoordinations

> . . . with the general lymph circulation have caused varied forms of toxic or dross conditions, used energies, to not be eliminated from the body. With the changing in glandular secretions and activities, there have come periods of general debilitation; not in the mental abilities of the body but physical debilitations, causing reflexes of a neuritic, arthritic nature—as in hands and feet and lower limbs at times. These become quite painful, and at other times are just heaviness, aching in those portions of the body.   3334-1

Fume baths (with witch hazel) followed by a thorough massage at least once a week for six to ten weeks were recommended. Dietary advice was also given. Unfortunately, no follow-up reports exist on her progress.

Aches and pains. These types of complaints are difficult to categorize adequately, especially since they can occur anywhere in the body—because pain receptors are abundantly distributed in the skin and deeper tissues—and originate from a variety of causes. For convenience, several cases presented in the readings on painful conditions are given here plus their relationship to the lymphatic system.

A twenty-eight-year-old man, who had four health readings from April to December 1943, asked, "What causes soreness in body, especially in lower abdomen and chest?" Four years earlier, he had suffered from chest colds, an upset stomach, and was coughing and wheezing. A severe cold in April 1943 prompted him to obtain another reading. In reply to his question, the reading stated:

> This is the effect of pressure upon the tissues of the body from those poisons or accumulations in the lymph, and these from plethoric conditions [excess of blood in the circulatory system] that produce pressures upon nerves through these areas, see? It is the liver, the kidney and the heart and lung circulation. Thus at times it will be as in the pit of the stomach, at others close around the heart, at others upon the right side high up, at others down across the lower portion of the abdomen, at others in the lower portions across the back.   568-4

Adjustments, massages, and castor oil packs were part of his regimen. At the end of the year in December, his mother reported that he had had convulsions in his sleep during the night. The previous October, he had fallen off a horse and received a concussion, causing a pressure on the right side of his head (according to reading 568-5). Several check readings helped him recover. In 1963 he quit his job at the navy shipyard and became a professional golfer. His first physical reading, 568-2, advised him that the exercise of golf would be excellent for him.

A thirty-year-old man, in his third and final reading, given on February 9, 1942, wondered about "the aches on the left side of my neck, also the little lumps." He was told: "These are a part of the effect from the lack of proper coordinating with the lymph circulation. And the character of treatments indicated—the hot and cold shower, a tub or sitz bath or both—will be beneficial." (2621-3) The reports following this reading note that he died on November 23, 1944, of Hodgkin's disease, as listed on his death certificate, with the onset of the disease occurring four years prior.

Neurasthenia, a virtually obsolete term, was the disorder that a twenty-seven-year-old woman was experiencing, characterized by depression and tired feelings throughout her body and legs; popularly, it was known as nervous prostration. She asked about the burning sensation in her left shoulder and her back. The reading stated that the cause was "the tendency for segments in this area of the spinal column to become clogged; thus preventing the proper flow of the lymph as well as the general nerve forces." (667-14) The reading acknowledged the strain on her nervous system, suggested some vitamin tablets, a diet of "body-building foods," and osteopathic adjustments. She had one more reading, which revealed a tendency toward tuberculosis and suggested use of the charred oak keg. By this time, late August of 1943, Cayce was booked up with appointments until September or October of 1944, so she did not schedule another reading; Cayce actually gave his final readings for others in August of 1944.

A pinching sensation in a "scar left by incision on my abdomen" was one seventy-eight-year-old woman's concern. There is no mention of the reason for the incision. The reading explained the pinching as "[t]he effect of the lack of lymph or the water blood supply, calling for activity and thus producing a drawing or the stitching, or pinching in these areas where excess of same has been necessary for resuscitating and building up body tissue." (851-4)

The bulk of the reading comprised her questions; only in one brief beginning paragraph did Cayce sum up her physical condition: many changes since her last reading (five years before), some as a result of "determined activity of mind," yet "toxic forces" were continuing to interfere with her overall health. She was delighted with the information in her reading, which also gave her hope, and continued to use castor oil packs on her liver. She kept up an active life until her death at age ninety. According to a note from her daughter, she attributed her good health to following Cayce's readings.

SPECIFIC BODY AREAS OR ORGANS

This next section covers difficulties related to certain organs or areas of the body in which the lymph played a role in their malfunctioning.

Head. Several people asked about the causes of their headaches. In a number of cases, improper lymph circulation with its resultant pressures contributed to this condition. One woman, suffering from occasional intense headaches, was told, " . . . this arises from the drying, or the overflowing of lymph; for these are pressures in the soft tissue of the antrum, and in the head and neck forces that produce same." (2072-9) She was advised to use the Violet Ray appliance during "these particular periods."

A twenty–four–year–old young man, through a verbal request from Helen Storey, member of Study Group #3, asked about his constant headaches and was told:

> The pressure of the lymph circulation upon those areas where there are the tendencies for sticking or adherence through the whole portion of the torso itself. There are tendencies for these to form into lymph tumors. Let's get away from this by the use of those things suggested.
>
> 533-9

When he asked what would relieve the headaches, he was told: "Taking sedatives and the like does *not aid*; it only produces a distressing condition. A gentle rub back of the head and along the spine is much preferable." (533-9)

Osteopathic manipulations, abdominal castor oil packs, and massages were recommended as well as an alkaline–reacting diet and Zilatone tablets to help drain the gall duct area and stimulate the liver. Earlier readings indicate a history of gastrointestinal inflammations. Surgeons wanted to operate, but his reading said he didn't need surgery if he followed the suggestions; he complied and an operation was avoided. Ten days after his reading, Helen Storey wrote:

> There is, a few doors from me now, a young man to whom five of the leading physicians in this city have told, "We have done all we can for you." This young man is well on the way to recovery. He knows and will

> gladly testify as to the wonderful benefit he received through the readings. He is most grateful and appreciative for the blessing that has been his through Mr. Edgar Cayce. 533-9, R-1

The young man eventually received twenty readings, his final one being a life reading; his brother and sister also received readings. In June 1963 he indicated that he "stays in fairly good health as long as he sticks to the diet and general treatments which were outlined for him in the readings." (533-19, R-6)

In the next two cases, conditions in the head related also to the stomach.

A fifty-one-year-old woman, who received a total of thirty-nine readings, asked in one physical reading about the tightness in her head. She had been experiencing vertigo, joint pain, blurred eyesight, and burning sensations in parts of her body. Some of these conditions, the reading stated, were due to an overacidity in her system. The tightness in her head was caused by "those centers in the dorsal area that have tightened up by the pressures, and that bringing to the *stomach* of an *acid* condition in the blood, and those forces in the *lymph* that make for that in the head and soft tissue of face—see?" (243-11)

The remedy suggested to clarify the head was "[t]he snuffing of Dobell's solution," a liquid consisting of sodium bicarbonate, borax, phenol, and glycerin; it was often used as a wash or spray for treating nasal and throat diseases and was recommended about a dozen times in other readings. She later developed intestinal problems, varicose veins (she was a milliner who stood a lot while waiting on customers), hypertension, a broken wrist, and a heart condition. Four years later, she still complained of headaches, resulting from dorsal pressures and poor circulation, but about a year later she was feeling better, having experienced a number of physical ups and downs. She died in 1957 in her seventies following removal of a stomach tumor.

Sinus conditions create headaches for a lot of people. One fifty-five-year-old gentleman, who from July to November 1931 received a total of four readings (several of them business related), asked about his sinus trouble and received this reply:

Did you ever see a time where Radium Water is given that they didn't
have this? These come from the lymph activities, which are more
effective in the soft tissues than most portions; though the condition
arises not from the sinus themselves, but is from the stomach, or from
that plexus in the *locomotion* that *gives* the activity to the soft tissue of
the face, the throat, the nostrils, and must—sooner or later—have its
effect upon the whole sympathetic nervous system, making for irritations to the general body, in that of becoming cross, irritated, easily
unbalanced—and the body wouldn't like that at all!   3861-1

Through the intervention of his nephew [279], Mr. [3861] requested
the reading, which contained questions regarding his business interests
as well as health concerns. A comment on the Radium Water was mentioned in the nephew's letter to his uncle: "I am certain, however, that if
you take the Radium Water, as he [Cayce] suggested, you will be cured
of any troubles you have been bothered with." (3861-1, R-1) Over a
dozen readings recommended Radium Water (which could be obtained,
according to reading 4601-1, from a company in Pittsburgh, Pennsylva-
nia: Radium Therapeutics) as a treatment for cancer and other various
disorders. The next reading for [3861] indicated that he had tendencies
toward diabetes and Bright's disease (a disease of the kidneys). No further reports exist on his condition or treatment success.

Hay fever, characterized by itching, watery eyes and sneezing, is a
common allergy, mostly in reaction to pollen and spores of molds. It
can cause inflammation of the ears, sinuses, throat, and bronchials.
Some hay fever sufferers may develop asthma. Avoiding the hay fever
season by vacationing in a pollen-free area may be one way of dealing
with this nuisance.

Mrs. [5148] believed that she was allergic to ragweed, had suffered
from this condition for a period of years, but found no treatments helpful. Both she and her husband received physical readings on May 25,
1944, and she asked about what to do to overcome her hay fever. The
reading responded:

In the correcting of the conditions in the coordination of the sympathetic
and cerebrospinal systems we will make the corrections necessary to

correct the circulation through the lymph flow to the soft tissue of head and throat. Thus the balance brought in the circulation and the eliminations through their channels should, for this body, eliminate the disorders.   5148-1

The formula for an inhalant was also given, the fumes of which would "act as an antiseptic and as an allayer of irritation." (5148-1) Follow-up questionnaires were sent out several times, but no reply was received. **Throat.** Several individuals had throat problems. One fifty-six-year-old woman whose blood condition indicated anemia was given a comprehensive treatment plan that the reading called "a campaign for the revitalization of the whole system . . . " (626-1) In addition to dietary advice and attitude changes, she was advised to use the charred oak keg, the Violet Ray appliance, carbonated or animated ash on her tongue, and to receive massages. Here was her throat complaint:

(Q) Please give cause for the difficulty I have at times in swallowing.
(A) Lack of the lymph circulation in those portions of the body that are affected . . . Hence the treatments from the violet ray, when those portions are taken, which will add to the oxygen for the system. About the third time, and we won't have much trouble with this.   626-1

This advice was added:

Do these things that we have outlined, in a consistent and persistent way and manner, and with that expectancy as we have indicated; knowing that all the necessary vital forces of the body may be applied and supplied from without, as all increase comes from the activative forces in the various forms of matter—as we have given—and we will find the body will begin, in at least three to five days, to find improvement.

626-1

Notations following the reading indicated that she "thought reading was wonderful; said so over and over; said she felt better already; said she would follow it in every detail." (626-1, R-1) However, no further information as to outcome exists.

Another woman, twenty-three years old, had a total of fifteen readings from Cayce from 1925 to 1942. She requested this check reading because she had just gotten over a dizzy spell and had lost some weight as a result. She asked about the origin of a choking sensation in her throat, especially when lying down, and the reading answered:

> The circulation attempting to balance itself through the activities of the extremities. As it rises toward the head through the central circulation, through those congested areas, it produces the choking sensation. An overflow of the lymph to the head.
>
> Follow the suggestions we have outlined, these conditions will be overcome; both as to the general health and as to those conditions from tendencies for cold and congestion.   421-8

She also had an anemic condition but began to carry out all the suggestions in the reading except for the inhalant, which she had difficulty getting a pharmacist to fill because of its alcohol content. She eventually struggled with a strep infection as well as tuberculosis and goiter tendencies. In 1952 her aunt reported that she had had five or six tumors removed—all benign—and came through the operation "like a trooper." (421-15, R-3) The last notation from her aunt revealed that [421] had been caring for her ill mother for the past fifteen months.

Another reference to a throat condition came not from a question presented by the recipient but in the reading's description of the physical condition of the person herself. She was told that a certain "fullness in the throat and bronchial" occurs at times because of "activities in the mucous or lymphatic circulation . . . not as a spasmodic, nor as other than a sympathetic nervous reaction." (3912-1) The present age of this female is not given, but the reading noted she had received a spinal injury during play when she was between eighteen months and two years old. No further references were made to her throat condition. Both she and her father were present for the reading.

A forty-eight-year-old sales manager (who received a total of 254 readings) requested a physical and business reading on January 15, 1942. One question concerned the dryness he was experiencing in his head and throat. The reading explained:

This is the attempt of the system to coordinate the necessity of lymph flow through the body. These are lymph pockets or glands that cause dryness. The salivary glands, the throat glands all are drawn upon to attend or to give better activity through other portions of the body; thus causing dryness. Closer adherence to the applications and activities suggested should keep such away from the body.   257-239

Then came this note of correction:

To have to continue to add properties to keep a balance, because of non-adherence to those first suggestions made, is not good—and is tempting the body and the better mental and physical interests of the body.   257-239

Earlier, his reading mentioned a drying effect throughout the alimentary canal and suggested "the occasional hydrotherapy and massage . . . so that the lymph flow is kept well, and that there be proper peristaltic movements in the muscular forces of the alimentary canal as a whole." (257–239)

The peristaltic movement referred to in this last extract is the process by which food, after being swallowed, is moved from the esophagus downward into the stomach and then, in smaller amounts, into the intestines, where further digestion takes place. The food waste eventually reaches the rectum, where it is discharged from the body. Muscular contractions in the walls of the digestive organs, in wavelike motions, move the food along and also aid in its disintegration, helping it mix with the digestive juices. Peristaltic waves are generally irregular, stronger sometimes and weaker at other times. They are also weaker in some individuals, especially the elderly.

Lungs. The two main organs of respiration, the lungs lie within the chest cavity behind the rib cage on either side of the heart. Their spongelike substance is made up of elastic tissue with networks of tubes, air sacs, and blood vessels. The right lung has three lobes, and the left two. Their main function is to transport oxygen received from the outside air into the blood and to remove carbon dioxide from the blood and expel it to the outside. The surface area of the lungs for this gas exchange is thirty times greater than the body's surface area (around 70 square meters, or 84 square yards, for an adult male). The action of the diaphragm, a large, dome-shaped muscle which forms the bottom of the thoracic cage, and the intercostal (between the ribs) muscles helps the lungs to inflate, while deflation is largely a passive movement involving the abdominal muscles. Air brought into the lungs is first filtered, warmed, and moistened, yet if the body's resistance is low, infectious organisms and other irritants can invade and cause disease.

One man was suffering the effects of bronchitis, which scarred his lungs so badly that physicians had given up on him and declared that he was in the last stages of tuberculosis. Yet "he wanted the reading to see if he could get well so as to care for his family." (572-1, B-1) He received nine readings between June 5, 1934, and April 24, 1935. In his fifth reading he asked if he had fluid in his left lung, and the answer came, "No. Rather is this the lymph that *gurgles* back." (572-5) He was also bothered by shortness of breath. Small doses of olive oil as well as beef juice, outdoor activities, and inhalations of brandy fumes were recommended along with an expectant attitude. He was also advised, "Do not allow a single day without an activity from the liver and kidneys to be near *normal*; for these are the balancing organs in the system." (572-5)

According to a notation made by Gladys Davis Turner, both he and his wife "were very pleased with 572-5, saying it was 'beautiful and splendid.'" (572-5, R-1) Unfortunately, he died a month after his last reading, on May 27, 1935. In reply to a questionnaire on September 16, 1940, his wife wrote: "Every time he had a reading it was perfect in its analysis of Mr. [572]'s condition. We followed the first few readings and he got great help. I believe he would have been living today if we had faithfully carried out the readings instead of putting him again into the hands of the doctors." (572-9, R-2)

The next case, for a thirty-eight-year-old woman [267], has to do with an anemic condition related to lymph. In her only health reading from Cayce, she asked outright:

(Q) What is the condition of the lymphatics?
(A) From any condition where there is anemia produced . . . either by

nerve shock or from the lack of sustaining forces in the system, the lymph is low. Hence the respiratory system should be considered, and the reactions from the use of such a respirator would be the best—and the instrument used by Crews is the only one you'll find any where near here, in this vicinity [Virginia]. 267-2

An osteopath, Gena Lowndes Crews worked briefly at the Cayce Hospital and was in charge of it shortly before it closed. She is mentioned in more than fifty readings. Besides adjustments and massages, she also administered colonics and a respiratory or lymph pump (advised in several other readings) to benefit the respiratory system. While no mention is made of [267]'s use of this instrument, she did have osteopathic treatments—at $2 a visit!—from Dr. Crews and derived improvement from them. Her reading also mentioned "incoordinations . . . that affect both the white *and* red blood supply and the lymph circulation." (267-2)

The same woman referred to earlier (see "Sensory Organs: Ears"), who had asked for help for the ringing in her ears, also wanted to know about a calcified "lump in my chest as large as a baseball. It has been diagnosed as a walled-off T.B. infection by some doctors and as a tumor by others. Can you tell me what it is? It has been there twenty-five years and does not seem to get any worse." (3334-1, B-1) Apparently, she was not troubled by it at all. The reading described it thus: "A glandular condition or a secretion of lymph that, with emunctory patches, has just accumulated. This should be dissipated. Do not bruise but dissipate, with the gentle massage and the oils." (3334-1)

Earlier in her reading, the fifty-one-year-old woman was given these detailed instructions on the massage, which also mentioned the lymph centers:

> Follow this [fume bath] with a thorough massage, in a rotary motion rather than pulling or beating, as to produce a real stimulation to the whole circulation—especially those centers where the emunctories and the lymph circulation coordinate with cerebrospinal, as well as where these are active forces through the torso and trunk portion of the body—just below the breast bone or the upper portion of this—just below the clavicle and through the whole area of the diaphragm, and then just

above the pubic center. Also massage on either side of the hips, at the
coordinating centers of the lymph circulation with the sciatic center in
the back portion of the hips and especially throughout the sacral.

3334-1

The massage oil formula consisted of Usoline or Nujol (6 ounces),
olive oil (1 ounce), peanut oil (2 ounces), oil of pine needles (1/2 ounce),
and liquefied lanolin (1/2 ounce). The ingredients were to be mixed in
the order named and the treatment given once a week for six to ten
weeks, left off for a while, then begun again. Unfortunately, no follow-
up reports exist on her results.

Stomach. Lying between the esophagus and the small intestine in
the alimentary canal, the stomach receives the partially digested food
and mixes it with its own secretions by peristaltic action. The food eventually reaches a consistency of thick soup and is gradually pushed into
the small intestine, where the digestion of food is completed. An average stomach holds about 1.5 quarts (1.4 liters) when full. It takes from
one to four hours for the stomach to become emptied of its digested
contents, depending upon the type and amount of food eaten.

In the Cayce readings, problems in the stomach that were related to
lymph include nausea, inflammation, gas, and pain. Twelve readings
refer to the stomach as the "medicine chest" of the body. (One reading
[3927-1] referred to the duodenum, a section of the small intestine, as a
"medicine chest.") A twenty-seven-year-old woman, dealing with the
aftereffects of anesthesia following pelvic surgery, was told that her nausea was due to the effects of an imbalance in the lymph and blood
supply. Taking cod liver oil and Codiron tablets "will build greater resistance, especially to the lymph and emunctory circulation—which is
needed to rid the system of the effects of those activities which were
given to suppress the nerve forces. For these tend to clog and clot
through the network as it were of the lymph and emunctories, especially." (263-10) A light steam bath to produce sweat, followed by a thorough massage, both taken about once a month, would help alleviate
the condition. After her next reading, she reported that she was now
following the suggestions and "I am very much better." (263-11, R-1)

In one man's physical reading, poor eliminations eventually resulted in "inflammation in the gastric flow." (294-194) The word *gastric* pertains to the stomach. This sixty-two-year-old had completed one day of a three-day apple diet but had discontinued because he was feeling so poorly. In this check reading he was advised to eat plain foods and no fruits. The condition, the reading stated, "may be called lymphitis," which technically would mean "inflammation of the lymph," though the term doesn't appear in the medical dictionary. Three months later, a follow-up reading indicated there was no inflammation, but the diet should still be adhered to along with outdoor activities and exercise.

One woman was given this description in her physical reading:

> In the pit of the stomach we find there are those accumulations that form gas, and these are from a plethoric condition in the lymph circulation, in the pyloric portion of the stomach itself. This, as we find, is an indication also of how, through incoordination between cerebrospinal and sympathetic nervous forces, which supply energies from brain and blood force by impulses, as well as the regular circulation which goes directed or controlled or influenced by this incoordination which exists here, there are produced segregations or accumulations which would be called tumorous in their nature.   5236-1

A plethoric condition means any excessive amount; in this case it was an overabundance of lymph.

The pyloric section lies at the distal end of the stomach, where it opens into the duodenum, the first portion of the small intestine. A fold of mucous membranes containing circular muscular fibers surrounds it, the ring of muscles opening and closing the aperture and passing the stomach's contents along to its next digestive phase.

In a letter one month before her reading, this forty-two-year-old woman expressed concern about a possible tumor in or near her uterus, also pains in the center of her body just above the lower ribs, as well as pain sometimes in her whole left side, including her arm and leg. In addition to dietary advice, regular massages and chiropractic treatments, the use of ultraviolet light with green glass, and colonics, the reading warned that surgery might be needed if the advice was not followed. No details on her physical health were reported in the follow-ups. Her sister, son, and niece also received readings.

A thirty–eight–year–old woman wondered what was causing "[t]he weakness and hurting inside my stomach." She had problems with dermatitis and had seen a skin specialist who "said the breaking out on my face and nose was a form of roseola." (513–2, B–1) Her skin was irritated and red at times, yet she stated, "I feel that the condition comes from some internal cause." The reading earlier noted a tendency throughout her body "for accumulations of lymph in pockets," particularly in the abdomen, the pelvic organs, and the colon, and stated further that "the general irritation as comes to most of the organs [arises] from those activities of the nervous system as well as the glandular system." (513–2) In answer to her question regarding her stomach pain, the reading reiterated its warning against taking strong laxatives "until the body is toned. The hurting is from the tendency of accumulations of lymph circulation into pockets along the system attempting to meet the needs owing to the poisons and the poor gland eliminations or activity and the poor eliminations from the alimentary canal." (513–2)

This physical reading, the only one she received, was given on June 10, 1937. Both she and her husband were present for it. She also had admitted to being highly nervous and requested some help with that. In August of 1940 in reply to a questionnaire, she wrote: "My entire physical condition is better. My nervous condition is much better. I rest better." Her mother had emergency surgery, so [513] neglected some of the suggestions, taking only half of the tonic and forgoing the spinal/hip massage, yet she concluded, "I am now much better in every way . . . " (513–2, R–1)

Mr. [257], a forty–eight–year–old sales manager whom we met earlier (see "Throat" section), requested a complete physical diagnosis, since it had been a year since his colon surgery to remove some polyps. The reading immediately predicted "greater disturbances" if he continued to ignore the warnings already repeatedly given to him. "There are no short cuts! One *must* meet self. It will not do to observe certain rules today and forget them tomorrow . . . " (257–232) After suggesting some remedies, Cayce asked for questions. The first one concerned the cause of "the constant annoyance or worry that appears in pit of stomach . . . " The explanation given was: "This . . . is the forming of pockets, or lymph pockets, in lacteal ends—by irritation, because of the unbalanced condition in the chemical forces generally of the body." (257-232)

According to *Gray's Anatomy*, "The lacteals are the lymphatic vessels of the small intestine, and differ in no respect from the lymphatics generally, excepting that they contain a milk-white fluid, the *chyle*, during the process of digestion, and convey it into the blood through the thoracic duct." (p. 623) Though [257] was feeling the disturbance in the stomach area, the cause lay farther in the GI tract, in the lacteals in the small intestine, with the appearance of lymph pockets "that may become infectious and form conditions that cause the drainage of blood through the stool, and thus become infected and again be very disturbing." (257-232) The subject of lymph pockets, their formation and treatment, is discussed in the next chapter. According to a follow-up reading (257-238), however, Mr. [257] was still bothered and concerned about these intestinal lymph pockets.

Small intestine. The body's main digestive organ, the small intestine is where food is chemically broken down for use in the body's cells. It comprises the longest section of the alimentary canal, averaging about 21 feet in length (nearly 7 meters) in the average person, extending between the stomach and the large intestine. Its three subdivisions are named the duodenum, the jejunum, and the ileum, which joins the large intestine at the ileocecal valve.

Only a small amount of food is processed at one time, while enzymes from intestinal cells and the pancreas plus bile from the liver help with the breakdown of food. The walls of the small intestine are well suited for its chemical function and are structured to increase the absorptive surface. Fingerlike projections called villi arise from the mucous membranes and are rich in capillaries and lacteals (modified lymphatic capillaries). Digested food is absorbed, then, through the inner lining of the mucosa cells into both the capillaries and the lacteals. Toward the end of the small intestine, the distal ileum, are increasing numbers of collections of lymphatic tissue in the submucosa referred to as Peyer's patches or glands. These patches attempt to confine infectious material (the undigested food residue at this point contains large numbers of bacteria) and prevent it from entering the bloodstream.

Because numerous references were made in the Cayce readings to specific components of the small intestine, they will be discussed separately in the next chapter.

Large intestine.   The final section of the digestive tract, about 6 feet in length (1.8 meters), is the large intestine, consisting of the ascending (right side) colon, transverse (across the middle) colon, the descending (left side) colon, and the sigmoid colon, which curves to the right and is connected to the rectum. Food contents are transformed from a liquid to a relatively solid state (feces) during the journey through this tube-shaped structure. Here water, vitamins, minerals, and electrolytes are absorbed from the fecal material. The intestinal glands, which are mucus-secreting, are not involved in the chemical digestion of food material; however, the numerous, but necessary, bacteria that inhabit the colon help further the digestive process by aiding in the body's absorption of nutrients.

A number of references in the readings address conditions of the large intestine, and several are mentioned here:

A fifty-eight-year-old man, whose son requested the reading, was given what turned out to be his final reading before his death two months later. He had been suffering from a liver and heart condition, and over a four-year period received a total of eight health readings. In reading 372-8 a question was asked about eliminations, and the answer included some information about corrective measures that had been and should be taken:

> ... there is the tendency to make for better circulation in the lymph and the emunctories throughout the intestinal tract. Hence these will make for the general tendencies to prevent the absorption of the muco-membrane activity through the general system.
>
> It will be necessary . . . that at times there be used eliminants or enemas, that the fecal forces may be carried from the system; or the feces, see? but the general tendency from the applications suggested is to create a better movement throughout the emunctory and lymph circulation, which *is* the activity that makes for the peristaltic movements throughout the intestinal system.
>
> Of course, with the enemas, there should be used the oil, or the agar, with the Glyco-Thymoline as an antiseptic, which tends to make a

relaxing of the colon without the deteriorating forces acting or setting up!
But the general conditions in the present arise from deteriorating of
the activities in the system, as to set up mortified activity in the system.
372-8

The above information mentions the connection between lymph activity and peristalsis, a relationship brought out several times in other
readings. The recommended laxative, agar, is a gelatinous product
extracted from seaweed and is used, as well, as a gelling agent in cooking.

Cayce in this reading seems also to have been in touch with the
seriousness of [372]'s condition. Several days after receiving notice of
[372]'s death, he sent a letter of condolence to the son, saying in part:

I know that no word that anyone could say can ease that pain that is felt
by one who feels so helpless in the face of suffering and death, but I just
want you to know that I feel from my own experience the loss that your
father's death has meant to you, and I am in hopes that your own
willpower and strength will come to your aid at this time. We know that
"God doeth all things well." We cannot question His ways. Suffering and
death [are] the lot of man. They are hard to face, but only in Him also
can we find strength . . .   372-8, R-4

An additional note concerns a question that was asked in the origi-
nal reading but left out by request:

(Q) Is this condition cancerous?
(A) Not cancerous. The cirrhosis produces tendencies that give much
of the appearance as of cancerous reaction, see? as also does the
condition that is active in destroying lymph and emunctory circulation,
or drying same.
    But, with the revivifying through electrical forces, through a stimula-
tion to the body, these conditions should disappear.   372-8, R-1

The term *cirrhosis* was what this reading described earlier as the medical name for [372]'s condition, stating that it was quite severe and in an

advanced stage, yet "[i]t will require persistence, patience, to combat these influences . . . " (372–8)

Another individual, Mr. [257], the sales manager mentioned earlier (see sections on "Throat" and "Stomach"), had had polyps removed from his colon and was bothered now by the scar. He asked in his reading, "Why does the left side above the incision sometimes feel a little sore?" The reading offered some understanding and consolation to those who have had abdominal surgery:

> This is a general condition that exists from contractions, or periods when through the intestinal system there are the needs for the discharging of accumulations that form in lymph pockets; which discharge takes place if there are the effective forces through the system. This is a sensitiveness that naturally arises in those who have had abdominal operation.
>
> 257-243

As noted earlier, the next chapter will include additional information on lymph pockets.

Mucus in the intestines is another condition that is addressed in the readings. While there is always a small amount of it present in the large intestine to help lubricate the passageway for fecal material, too much mucus can inhibit peristaltic movement, resulting in a sluggish colon in which inflammation from toxic buildup can occur. One person, forty-seven–year–old [264], asked directly what was the cause of the "mucous condition in intestines" and what could she do to correct it. In reply, the reading gave a fuller explanation of the lymph function:

> . . . there should be added sufficient of the elements and forces that will produce a greater or better lymph circulation. You see, it is in the activity through the body, especially in throat, lung and intestines especially, that the greater portion of the circulation is carried on; through what may be called the *sympathetic* or the superficial circulation—and is of the lymph and emunctory nature.
>
> Then, when there is a deficiency in the blood stream to such an extent that it impoverishes especially those portions of the system, there comes the inclination for accumulations in such measures and man-

ners. For the activity of the lymph is to pass through the organ itself, as it were, as is necessary through the activity of the whole of the intestinal tract.

While there are ducts and glands and lymph throughout, both internally and externally, when these become impoverished by the lack of circulation in same it produces an inflammatory condition which through the stool would indicate mucous—sometimes even bloody conditions, see?   264-55

The importance of lymph circulation is stressed along with its reliance on an adequate working relationship with the blood. The answer continued, explaining the preponderance of the lymph pathways:

Hence if we would build up the resistances in the blood stream by a greater quantity of lymph, these will take on the lymph first—for it is the white portion or the watery portion. Lymph flows through the lymph ducts and lymph glands, and is a part of the whole nerve circulation. Hence in the superficial portions it expresses or manifests itself in networks over all portions of the abdomen, through the groin, and works through those activities along the mammary glands and salivary glands, and all portions of the alimentary canal.   264-55

"Lymph . . . is a part of the whole nerve circulation." (264–55) This is certainly an interesting comment from a medical standpoint of the lymph's status, or rank, in the human body. While lymph is generally associated with either the circulatory or the immune system, the words "nerve circulation" imply a diffusion or conduction of some type of electrical energy by which various parts of the body may communicate with one another, adding another dimension to its transportation function.

CONCLUSION

Describing and explaining the body section by section may be a more manageable way to present the activity of the lymphatic system. Yet, as a reminder, the wholeness of our physical selves is a consideration as well, enabling us to function as one, though with many parts. The next chapter presents the influence of the lymph in a more systemic fashion, taking into account several areas, organs, or sections that are affected and influenced by lymph activity.

CHAPTER FIVE

· · · · · · · · · · ·

Systemic Conditions Related to Lymph

The term *systemic,* of course—as its name implies—refers to systems, in this instance, bodily or physical systems. Anything that affects the body as a whole is considered "systemic." The opposite meaning would be "local." Several examples of the latter are what were described and mentioned in chapter 4. Earaches, painful areas, hay fever, a sore incision, or the swelling of a lymph node or a slightly infected wound are some conditions of local trouble. However, if the local defenses are breached, a larger response is called for to contain the spreading infection, resulting in signs of fever or a high white blood cell count, for now it has reached global (or systemic) proportions, affecting more body areas.

The Cayce readings, no doubt, with their comprehensive overview of bodily systems and how they holistically function and operate in an integrative manner, present a unique way of dealing with illness and disease. Each physical reading, given for and offered to a particular individual, also has a quality of uniqueness about it. Yet there is retained an air of universality in these physical readings that invites participation from others with similar stresses and concerns. While a certain reading will, of course, not be identical to another particular person's, yet a common bond somehow may be felt, and a desire to carry out its treatments may follow.

One visitor to A.R.E. expressed it this way. He was fascinated by psychics and, following this interest, had been doing a study of them, researching their readings, finding out all that he could about each of them. So he came to Virginia Beach to the A.R.E. headquarters to pursue his interest in the Cayce perspective. So, from all the information that he had gathered, how did Cayce compare as a psychic with the others he had researched? His comment was:

> When I read an individual's report from another psychic, I think, Yes, that reading fits that person exactly. It's really right on for him or her. But when I read through a Cayce reading, I know it's meant for a particular person, but *I* get something out of it, too! There seems to be oftentimes a message or statement that I can apply and use, that has meaning *for me*, though I know it's from another person's reading. From no other psychic do I get that kind of feeling or response.

In one sense, this impression of the A.R.E. visitor resembles the difference between a local and a systemic condition, the "local" being the meaning for that particular person who requested the reading and "systemic" being a more comprehensive meaning from which others may derive benefit. A relevant addendum to this comparison is a comment frequently made by Gladys Davis Turner, Edgar Cayce's longtime secretary: this body of information contains nothing new; it's material we've always known, but Cayce is simply bringing it to our remembrance, helping us to recall or perhaps re-remember what we've always known but have forgotten. This perspective may help to explain the familiarity people experience when they first encounter the readings. Despite the convoluted sentences and rather archaic language they must wade through, a meaningful message comes across, nevertheless, something that seems applicable and helpful to the one perusing the reading.

In this vein, then, the following section presents more detailed explanations of the physical conditions of the recipients, with regard to the nature of their particular health condition. It offers a thumbnail sketch of several health concerns that involve the lymphatic system, but more extensive than previously presented. Because of space limitations, however, only a few representative cases are given below.

CONDITIONS RELATED TO ORGANS OF ELIMINATION

Kidneys and bladder.   Ordinarily, people have two kidneys, each with a ureter, a tube that drains urine from the kidneys into the bladder. From the bladder, then, urine drains through the urethra and out of the body. The primary function of the kidneys is filtering the metabolic wastes and excess sodium and water from the blood and eliminating these products from the body. In a twenty–four–hour period 40 gallons (150 liters) of water are filtered out from the blood by the kidneys; about 99 percent is returned, with 3 pints (1.5 liters) forming urine. The kidneys are also involved in red blood cell production and help regulate blood pressure.

The term *hepatic*, mentioned in the next excerpt, appears more than two thousand times in the readings; according to the dictionary, it refers to the liver. Yet, in the Cayce readings, the kidneys, bladder, heart, and lungs were also included as part of the hepatic circulation, sometimes described as upper and lower hepatic circulation, with several of these organs included in one or the other.

In the seventh Cayce reading for a forty–eight–year–old woman, her "tendency towards constipation in the hepatic circulation" was described as a "lack of lymph to carry on proper incentives from those centers from which there is carried on the radiation of activity." (243-7) What an unusual choice of words in the earlier phrase—"constipation in the hepatic circulation"—since the term *constipation* has to do with difficult or infrequent evacuation of fecal material from the large intestine. Perhaps this is how the Cayce source chose to describe what he saw occurring in [243]'s circulatory system. The reading earlier had been pointing out the correlation that exists between the blood and the lymph circulation and went on to explain in more detail the nature of insufficient lymph, in the process offering a fuller understanding of the purpose and work of the lymphatic system:

The lymph we find being the secretions of the body that oil or supply elasticity to the whole system, in its activity in any functioning organ of the body. When there is a lack of this, distress or distraughtness comes to the portion thus affected. Not so much that the body is carrying poisons back, though it is that of an ash—or non-elimination, but there is the lack of sufficient lymph to carry on through that center—by the hindered capillary circulation.   243-7

This action, the reading continued, was producing her tendency toward hepatic constipation. Again, an improper or insufficient flow of lymph, needed to "oil or supply elasticity to the whole system," was creating problems or distresses in her body. She received a total of thirty–nine readings (see also her brief accounts under "Bones: Knots" and "Specific Body Areas: Head" in chapter 4) and suffered physical ups and downs throughout her life, dying in 1957 in her seventies.

That our bodies work hard at self–correcting is expressed repeatedly throughout the health readings. Oftentimes while this process is being carried out, we may experience other discomforts that, unbeknownst to us, are directly related to the systemic condition that has been developing over time, like a domino effect. Such was the case with Mrs. [243]. The reading explained it carefully, then added a comparison to elucidate it further:

There is congestion, then, in the liver. The kidneys become involved by too much being thrown on the kidneys to eliminate. Hence, whenever there is scarcity of the secretions through the secreting system, we have these distresses appearing through the lower portion of the back, or along that same region in which there is the tie-up in cerebro-spinal as well as sympathetic system, and pains across the back, through the right and left sides. Each of these shows that all of the system, attempting to come to the aid of the body in its attempt to eliminate, produces distresses on the body. It is not an organic condition, though—without correction—it may become so; that is:

Just as a comparison—of a poor nature, but—a rotten apple left in a barrel may make all of these rotten; yet no matter how many sound ones are put about it, the rotten one will never be made sound.
                                                            243-7

Notice that one of the "distresses" she was experiencing was low back pain. One A.R.E. colon therapist some time ago had an episode of low back pain that seemed difficult to heal. She had steams, massages, Reiki, and packs, but the pain persisted. Finally, she received a colonic and, lo and behold, the pain disappeared! Believing initially that the origin of the pain was muscular, she had tried various treatments; however, the pain was referred from her congested colon and the colonic relieved it. Now, she says, whenever she has an episode of low back pain, she knows just the treatment to undertake.

A few weeks before her seventh reading, Mrs. [243] wrote in a letter that she had a reoccurrence of neuritis (nerve inflammation) as well as constant headaches, swollen hands and feet, and a burning sensation throughout the veins in her thighs, feet, and hands. "I feel sometimes like fire is on the inside of my skin." (243-7, B-2) Her physician said that her kidneys were to blame, and in her confirmation letter acknowledging the next reading appointment, she mentioned her swollen veins and stated, "I really believe my kidneys are affected, but can you find out for me." (243-7, B-3) This seventh reading, then, quoted in part earlier, was taken on December 19, 1927; three months later, she also received a check reading. She seemed to have difficulty following her readings consistently, experiencing a number of successes and failures in her efforts.

In a reading given on November 26, 1930, for a six-year-old, [2373], whose mother requested this one and only reading, a question was asked if he had an infection or inflammation in his bladder. According to a previous question, [2373] had been frequently passing water. The reading answered that no infection, but inflammation, was present, "produced by the excessive amount of the lymph pressure in system attempting to be eliminated through these channels." (2373-1) Because the question had also included "what is the cause and remedy," the answer concluded:

> When we have cleansed the colon, and have had antiseptic reactions through the intestinal system—and relieved those pressures in the lumbar and cervical regions—we will find a better coordination established in eliminations, and drainages and eliminations set up through

their *nominal* channels—rather than through the weakened conditions
in the impulses to the organs' functioning—will bring near normalcy.

2373-1

As in the majority of Cayce's health readings, there was offered the
possibility of cure for the condition, in this instance through the use of
enemas and osteopathic adjustments. Earlier in [2373]'s reading, he was
told that there were "disturbances in the nerve system" that could be
detected "by the very nature of the blood stream itself; for the lymph
and the emunctories show the effect of a nerve disturbance." This disturbance was manifesting "in the burses as are seen in the extremities
. . . a soreness as results from same . . . " This was not rheumatism, the
reading said, nor "even an *elementary blood* disorder, though the blood
becomes *involved*" simply because of its distribution. A bursa (plural,
bursae) is a fluid-filled sac that provides extra cushioning between adjacent areas, such as between bones and tendons, that otherwise might
rub against each other, causing pain as well as wear and tear. An increase in the amount of lymph was also creating "improper coordina-
tions in burse centers," affecting the digestive system and mental reflexes,
resulting in "regurgitation throughout the activities of an *assimilating*
system." However, the reading stated that this was not the cause but
rather a reflex condition. Because of incoordinations in the cervical
(neck) region, impulses to the body (received from the lymph ducts and
glands) were irritating "the throat, head, and the *sensory* system . . . all of
the *sensory* organisms." (2373-1)

Though [2373]'s mother requested the reading, there is no background
information submitted as to what were this boy's health concerns. From
comments and questions in the reading, there are descriptions of [2373]'s
tendencies to arthritis as well as some nervous, jerky movements that
occurred from time to time. While information outside of the reading
itself is virtually nonexistent, there is one final statement from the boy's
uncle, reporting in September 1975 that the boy's parents did not follow
through with the recommendations in his reading.

A forty-three-year-old marble worker, Mr. [779], requested his twentieth reading because of severe pain in his lower back and hips. The
reading was categorized under "lumbago" and referred to pain in the

lumbar region of the back. (In another reading, 404-7, Cayce described lumbago as "the effect of uric acid in portions of the eliminating system . . . " resulting, in this person's case, from an acute muscular condition owing to "the effect of incoordination between the upper and lower hepatic circulation . . . " (Uric acid is a waste product present in blood and excreted in the urine.) The reading immediately pointed out specific areas needing attention:

> There is a lack of those vital forces in the activity of the glands themselves, as related to the functioning of the tissue or minutia in the lymph circulation, through the eliminating forces in the kidneys in the whole hepatic circulation. Hence those disorders, or distresses, where circulation has been hindered in the extremities.   779-20

Poor circulation caused him to have cold hands and feet, and the information reminded him that "[t]hese are but signs of the conditions, and are the results of those disorders in the lymph circulation through the intestinal system, as related to the hepatic circulation." Next followed a listing of the resultant effects: muscles contracted, dizziness, a drumming in the ears, a need to clear the throat, blurry eyes, and "improper distribution of blood supply through the head and neck, face, eyes . . . " Hot salt packs placed across the lower back, Atomidine, the Violet Ray machine, and exercise were all recommended as part of his regimen. "These . . . will aid the body in gaining its *normal* equilibrium, ridding the system of those infectious forces as attacked the emunctory and lymph circulation—especially through those of the lower hepatic circulation." (779-20)

Two weeks later, [779] stated, "I am feeling lots better and think in a short while I will be 100% again." (779-20, R-1)

CONDITIONS RELATED TO ORGANS OF DIGESTION

Small intestine. The longest and most convoluted section of the GI tract, the small intestine is where the digestion of food is completed, the digested food—called chyme—being absorbed through its walls into the bloodstream, while the undigested portion is passed along to the large intestine. Essentially all nutrients, including vitamins, are digested in the small intestine, and up to 95 percent of fats and 90 percent of amino acids, which are protein building blocks, are absorbed.

There are three subdivisions of the small intestine: a short upper portion, the duodenum (10 inches; 25 centimeters); the central jejunum (8 feet; 2.5 meters); and the final two–thirds, the ileum (about 12 feet, or 3.5 meters). Lymphatic and blood capillaries located in and about the villi, finger–shaped projections that protrude from the folded inner surface of the walls, are where nutrients of molecular dimensions are absorbed. Muscles in the walls of the small intestine contract rhythmically, moving the food along and swirling it around to bring it into better contact with these absorbing cells. These nutrients, which pass into the blood and lymph vessels of the wall, are eventually transferred to the rest of the body. To get an idea about how extensive this inner layer is, if its surface were laid out flat, it would be about 2¼ miles (3.6 kilometers) long.

In summary, then, in the small intestine, most of the digestion of food (in the chemical sense) takes place, and the products of digestion are absorbed into the blood and lymph. Smooth muscle contractions facilitate these processes as well as move along unabsorbed food residues and other excretory products into the large intestine. The villi that line the small intestine are rich in lymph vessels called lacteals, which run up the center of each villus and are filled with lymph fluid. They are also especially important in the absorption of fat, a rich source of energy for the body.

Lacteals are mentioned more than one thousand times in the readings, and their role in absorption was often pointed out. The readings also referred to them as "glands of assimilating" (2096-2) or "the assimilating center of the system itself" (4675-1). Another reading described them as "cords in the intestinal tract through which there is the absorption of that assimilated into the circulation." (257-217) According to Dr. Harold Reilly, the term *assimilation*, as Cayce used it, involves "the individual's capacity to utilize the food and the body's performance of the complicated metabolic processes of digestion and elimination of indigestible material." (p. 27) In other words, how well your body utilizes the nutrients from the food you have eaten or the process by which it transforms that food into living tissue—that is what is meant by assimilation, considered one of the pillars (the A in the CARE acronym) of good health.

A problem in the lacteals was mentioned in the case of a thirty-two-year-old woman who received her only reading on August 26, 1942, and was present during it. She had been having longtime abdominal pain; however, the technical diagnosis of her condition, as stated by her osteopath, Dr. George Coulter, in a written report on January 14, 1943, was "chronic naso-pharyngeal catarrh." (2797-1, R-4) She presented a number of complaints—including menstrual cramps, numbness in her foot and leg, a rash on her forehead—and had been going to doctors and sanitariums for fifteen years, trying to get relief. Here is the question and answer from her reading mentioning the lacteals:

> (Q) Why do I always have a pain and a heavy feeling in the right side of my abdomen?
> (A) Because of the lymph activity through the digestion, as we have stressed here. This is the area from which there is the distribution from the activity of the lacteals. And there are pressures caused there from the drawing on this area for lymph flow through other portions of the body. Hence, as indicated, do not take fats—that is, fats in meats or great quantities of butter or of sweets, especially during the periods of these treatments [hydrotherapy, osteopathic adjustments, massages]. And with the massage, when the body is thoroughly relaxed, this should be a part of the treatment; kneading, gently, the upper abdomen. For, as indicated, this irritation through the jejunum is a part of this heaviness in the right side.   2797-1

So elimination of fats from her diet would help relieve the pressures in the lacteals. Other readings for different individuals mentioned also not only pressures in the lacteals but congestion, repression, adhesions, clogging, or accumulations, as well as acid conditions—all of which would throw the body out of balance. To aid in correcting these conditions of imbalance, in addition to dietary advice, were suggestions for hydrotherapy treatments, osteopathic manipulations, colonics, and various medicinal or herbal supplements, all of which were also prescribed for Mrs. [2797].

Her reading reflected the condition of the so-called domino effect, with pressures in her third and fourth cervical vertebrae affecting the face and soft tissue in her throat and head. "In the throat and nasal passages there is produced an extra flow of lymph that is active in the mucous membranes. This becomes infectious from the lack of the proper flow, or the hormones in the blood itself, or the white or lymph blood." (2797-1) A swelling in those areas—face, throat, and head—occurred as a result of her body's attempt to adjust itself. "The flow of lymph from these [areas] causes a reaction in the digestive forces, and this continues as a vicious cycle of nerve tensions to the body." (2797-1) Her eliminatory organs became involved as a result, with muscular contractions ("of the peristaltic movement") throughout her small and large intestines—a reflex action, the reading stated, because of "the lymph disturbance."

Schematically, the effect could be summarized thus: vertebral pressures → swelling in face → infection → digestion affected → "nerve tensions" → "eliminations . . . involved." Relief was possible "if there is the systematic reaction given the body forces as to aid in bringing normal impulses through the body." She was likewise encouraged "to be an expression for a manifestation of a purpose for good, for God, in the earth." (2797-1)

Her doctor's reply to a questionnaire stated that he felt the reading correctly described the condition, the suggestions seemed appropriate, and that he had treated [2797] osteopathically twice a week for six weeks. As far as results, he wrote, "The condition improved and the patient felt more comfortable." However, her move to Washington, D.C., resulted in a discontinuation of the treatments with him; yet he added a further comment: "This case would have gotten permanent relief, I believe, if treatment had been continued." Unfortunately, no further follow-up account exists.

Peyer's Patches. Referred to briefly in chapters 2 and 4, Peyer's patches (or glands) are named after a Swiss doctor, Johann Konrad Peyer, who in 1677 described these oval areas of lymphatic tissue in the small intestine. Found only occasionally in the jejunum, they are the most characteristic feature of the ileum, the terminal two-thirds of the small intestine. These small patches, from 1 centimeter wide to 5 centimeters long (1 cm=0.39 inch), are aggregates of lymph nodules that help to confine infectious material and prevent bacteria from penetrating the intestinal wall and entering the bloodstream. These patches are ideally located to capture and destroy bacteria, which are always present in tremendous numbers in the intestine, and act as a sentinel from the constant attacks of foreign material. Thus, they play an important role in the body's fight against infection, manufacturing large numbers of lymphocytes, key cells in our immune system, to repel the microscopic invaders. With age, the patches tend to get smaller and may even be destroyed by certain diseases, such as typhoid fever. One reading states:

> Hence the poisons, or the seat of the condition where poisons are absorbed in the system, being in the small intestinal tract, near the region of the Peyer's Patches or Peyer's Glands. This then is the seat of the conditions to be treated and corrected. 4326-1

No doubt because of its function of preventing bacteria from being absorbed in the body, the readings emphasized its importance to the health and well-being of the entire person, although today we still don't fully understand this role. References to Peyer's glands or patches occur in more than sixty readings, several of which, as in 4326-1 above, point to its dysfunction as the "seat" of the trouble for the whole system.

In *The Oil That Heals: A Physician's Successes with Castor Oil Treatments*, author William A. McGarey, M.D., addresses the role of Peyer's patches in the overall health of the individual, believing "that [from the Cayce perspective] the health of the nervous system was, to an extent, maintained through the substances that the Peyer's patches elaborate when they—the patches—are in good health." (p. 89) He mentions that a balance or "perfect contact between the sympathetic and cerebrospinal nervous systems [is] made possible through substances created in these small patches of lymphatic tissue in the mucosal surface of the small intestine . . . " These substances, then, are carried through the lymphatics and blood supply to the ailing portions of the nervous system. This exciting concept, he added, "leads us to wonder just what part these patches play in the physical disturbances that come about when we are subjected to stresses and worries that we hold on to in our minds and the emotional parts of our bodies." (p. 91) In other words, it seems that the Cayce readings relate the overall health of an individual directly to the healthy state of the Peyer's patches. We can only wonder about the correctness of this concept since, as mentioned earlier, their function today is not well understood.

On September 22, 1924, an adult female requested and was present for a reading, given in Dayton, Ohio. No background information or reports describe her presenting complaint, and there were no questions asked in the text of the reading. In beginning the reading, the Cayce source even stated, "Now this body we find very good throughout, and in many respects an exceptional body from the mental and spiritual side of the entity." (4870-1) Her two main problems, as determined from the reading, seemed to be poor eliminations and some spinal subluxations. The impingements in her lumbar (lower back) area were giving her a "tingling, deadening, sensation, to the lower or under part of arms, elbows, finger tips . . . " It was also affecting her hips and the arches of her feet.

> Digestion better than it has been and functions fairly normal . . . The disturbance then being in the Peyer's glands region, that is, the Peyer's Patches in the small intestinal tract. With these being and giving the supply of the system to carry on intestinal digestion, these not functioning normal allow poisons to be absorbed in system.   4870-1

The reading suggested osteopathic and chiropractic manipulations and predicted it would take six to eight treatments (if done correctly) to alleviate the disturbance. A formula for an herbal tonic was also given, two teaspoons twice a day before each morning and evening meal. No records exist as to the outcome.

Two separate readings recommend remedies that directly affect these glands. In one, 760-2, small doses of olive oil, taken by mouth often throughout the day for easier assimilation, as a food "as well as a lubri–cant . . . is an active property for duodenum, liver and upper portion, especially in the region . . . of the Peyer's Patches or Glands." The reading also mentioned that the pure olive oil would relax the condition in the small intestine in addition to relaxing the reaction that could occur in other areas of the GI tract.

In a second reading, gentle massage to the region of the Peyer's patches was suggested to aid in "preventing inflammation [from] setting up in specific places, and so thinning the walls of intestines as to cause rupture." (4313-3) The small intestine is located fairly centrally in the abdomen, around and below the navel, with the ileum, the section of the small intestine where the majority of these patches are located, slightly to the right side of the abdomen. This would be the region of concentration for the recommended abdominal massage.

Large intestine.   Roughly 6 feet (1.8 meters) in length, the large intestine is where the undigested food is moved along and eventually expelled from the body. Also called the bowel, it extends from the ileum (the end of the small intestine) to the anus and consists of three divisions: the ascending colon (on the right side of the abdomen), the transverse colon (lying across the middle of the abdomen), and the descending colon (the left side of the abdomen). Where the ileum joins the large intestine is the ileocecal valve, through which food passes from the small intestine into the large intestine. Unlike the small intestine, the large intestine has no villi or permanent folds in its walls. It does have cells that absorb water and inorganic salts, which are transported to the blood and lymph systems; other cells secrete mucus to lubricate the colon's contents. Bacteria, which inhabit the large intestine, aid in further digestion, manufacture vitamin K and several B vitamins, and are necessary for healthy intestinal function.

Constipation.   Not a true disease, constipation is a symptom common to a number of people who experience difficulty in passing stools or have infrequent or incomplete eliminations. Since ancient times, enemas and cathartics (medicines that stimulate bowel evacuation, also known as purgatives) have been used to purge the intestines. Native Americans used a combination of herbs and magic potions, while bowel specialists in ancient Egypt, as early as 2500 B.C., cleared the intestines with a variety of fluids, including ox bile. The Chinese Hippocrates, Chang Chung Chin, back in A.D. 196 preferred enemas over cathartics for their efficiency and ease on the body's system. The Greeks used water or saline solutions as enemas, a combination which is more medically correct.

Opinions on how often healthy people should have a bowel evacuation vary widely, ranging from two to three times a week to several
times a day. Regular times for elimination are important, since fecal
matter becomes hard, dry, and difficult to pass if it remains too long in
the colon. Diet and exercise are also important components to regular-
ity. The readings, while at times recommending laxatives, do not heart-
ily endorse them, as they can create a dependency upon them and may
inhibit the defecative reflexes, thus even causing constipation.

In a letter written to Cayce dated May 16, 1943, a thirty–two–year–old
woman requested help for her bruised right hip, which she had injured
nearly nine years previously. Her written account relates the incident
which caused the injury, one of those seemingly accidental events that
occurs to many of us at one time or another. In her case it involved
brother and sister pulling off each other's heavy riding boots. Here is
her narrative:

> Almost nine years ago, on July 26, 1934, I pulled off my brother's riding
> boots, and in doing so I injured my right hip. My brother put his foot on
> my right hip and the small of my back and pushed with the right boot
> on, while he had me straddling his left leg and pulling the left boot off,
> which was stuck from having been on since 6 a.m. to about 11 p.m. that
> night. So it was a strenuous struggle and terrific pull for me. The other
> boot I pulled off my way, facing him from the front, and pulling.
>
> I was in bed for six months afterwards, and it was a year before I could
> sit up without severe pain. Then it was years before I felt anywhere near
> normal again, a very slow recovery to normalcy. I have to wear a special
> corset for support with steel bones up the back, for what the doctors say
> was a sacro-iliac condition. It's better, but I'm still restricted in activity—
> have to be careful not to strain or hurt it, and walk only so much, and
> can't pull a car door, lift anything too heavy, or lie in bed on the right side
> more than a few minutes when it's feeling stronger.
>
> I've slept on my back entirely ever since July 26, 1934. My left side
> hurt too after that, but got well. Then the heart condition developed,
> which prevented resting on the left side either. It would be a blessing
> from God if the trouble could be fully and completely corrected.
>
> 3076-1, B-1

She had seen a chiropractor, but "his treatment only aggravated and increased the pain tenfold. He, undoubtedly, didn't know what the proper treatment should be. Please try and help me, Mr. Cayce." She submitted questions regarding her leg pains, chronic constipation, and poor vision. She received her one and only reading on July 6, 1943.

Early on, her reading pointed out an insufficient lymph circulation in the region, that is, not enough lymph moving "through the area to prevent a stiffness, or to keep from some deterioration—that has come through the years." (3076-1) The information also indicated "some lack of proper assimilation through the digestive area" that was due to an imbalance "between the alkalines and acids."

When she asked about relief from her chronic constipation, which had bothered her since she was a baby, the Cayce source replied:

> This, again, is a part of this circulation through the alimentary canal in the lymph. And the increasing in the amount of the character of food indicated, as well as the massage, should materially aid. Rather than too much of cathartics, use enemas—or colonic irrigations. These even taken once each month (the colonics), or twice each month at times, will be found to be helpful.   3076-1

Earlier, the reading suggested more seafood in her diet, which would increase her iodine and calcium intake. She was also to have a weekly "massage—osteopathically given."

In a follow-up letter, she questioned Cayce about the massage. One osteopathic doctor told her that he did only manipulations, not massage ("which would never correct anything"). (3076-1, R-1) Cayce answered in his letter to her:

> An osteopath can give a massage which is a certain type of osteopathic treatment. However, I know Dr. S. a little better, but I know he has handled several cases that we have given readings for. I do hope that you can take advantage of this.
>
> ... Thanking you, and be sure to let me know what you decide and who gives you the treatment. Hoping to have been the means of being of a real service ...   3076-1, R-2

For her poor vision, the reading recommended the head–and–neck exercises. No reports indicate the outcome of these treatments.

Often the readings, when describing the status of one's lymphatic system, would refer to the drying effect that was occurring, meaning an insufficient flow of lymph or some type of sluggishness or inactivity that creates a reduction in lymph circulation. Such was the case with [869]. A thirty–five–year–old male, he had had an ulcer and was suffering from gas and chronic constipation. The exploratory nature of the reading noted a catarrhal condition in his system (which was affecting blood and lymph flow) and congestion in his upper respiratory tract. The acidity of his system was influencing his digestion, causing gas as well as inflammation of the mucous membranes. An alkaline diet was suggested.

As for his chronic constipation, the reading stated it was due to "the lack of the flow of the gastric [stomach] forces through the jejunum." (869-1) This would be alleviated with "better peristaltic activity throughout the eliminating system" by having adjustments to the lower dorsal and lumbar spine as well as following a specific diet: less starch and sweets; more nuts, raw vegetables, and fruit; little meat; no fried foods. Then this clarification was added:

> When there is the tendency for inflammation or infectious reaction in lymph and emunctory activity in the mucous membranes of the body, this produces a drying condition and the lack of activity through the muscular forces of the intestinal system.   869-1

In such cases a type of stimulant is needed; for [869], use of diathermy was recommended as a form of electrotherapy that in his case was not to contain too high a voltage; it would "stimulate to nearer normal activity." (869-1) Used in conjunction with spinal manipulations, the treatment was advised to be taken twice a week for up to eight to ten times, then he was to rest and then resume the schedule.

Diathermy is mentioned in more than one hundred readings. Its purpose is to produce heat in the body, thus having a number of beneficial effects. *An Edgar Cayce Home Medicine Guide* states: "The Edgar Cayce readings often referred to diathermy as 'deep therapy.' In 46% of the cases researched, emphasis was placed on using a current of low frequency while 20% mentioned what could be termed low power." (p. 44) Evidently, both the long- and short-wave methods were readily available in Cayce's day.

In a number of readings there appears to be a link between the condition of the lymph and an increase or decrease in peristaltic activity. Peristalsis is the wavelike, rhythmic movement throughout the walls of the alimentary canal which moves the food, the contents of the tube, forward and onward. Muscles in the walls contract and dilate in an alternate manner, pushing the food to its proper destination. One reading states emphatically: "For it is the lymph flow that makes for activity through the alimentary canal, and when there is the tendency for the inflammation (not necessarily just irritation, but *inflammation*), it produces, of course, the drying of the lymph flow." (1140-2) Regular colonics using a saline solution, a few drops of olive oil taken internally three to five times daily, and an abdominal massage with olive oil, as much as the body would absorb, were the suggested treatments.

Though another statement was in reference to a swollen stomach, the reading, after advocating a massage "across the body," mentioned that such a treatment "should work up the peristaltic movement—which, of course, is the activity of the lymph and emunctory connecting forces of the intestinal tract itself." (1594-2)

Acidic conditions may also determine the status of one's peristaltic activity, as this reading notes: "As acids make for easy congestion either from cold or from the effects that are created by cold, there are periods when constipation is produced through the alimentary canal—or the *lack* of the flow of the lymph to carry on the proper peristaltic movement through those actions of the ascending colon." (668-1)

Temperature and lack of exercise and movement could also be factors in affecting lymph flow. Note this question-and-answer exchange:

(Q) [Why the] Seeming obstruction in intestines?
(A) Lack of sufficient lymph flow and the slowing of the general peristaltic movement, which arises either from inactivity or from temperature using up the lymph and emunctory forces; thus making less leucocyte activity in same as a motivative force through general activity in the intestinal system.   851-4

Awareness of these mitigating factors may lead us to be more obser-
vant of our intestinal system as it processes our nutrients and elimi-
nates our waste products in an efficient and timely manner. Proper diet
and regular exercise also play roles in maintaining a healthy intestinal
environment.

ANOTHER SYSTEMIC CONDITION RELATED TO LYMPH

Fever. While not necessarily a harmful condition, an increase in temperature does often alert the ill person that one's body is fighting an
infection somewhere. Elevation of body temperature is thus a protective response that enhances the body's defense. Other causes of fever
may stem from allergic reactions, hormone imbalances, inflammation,
excessive exposure to heat, or undiscovered cancer. That the lymph is
implicated in some of these conditions is not surprising, taking into
account its immune and infection-fighting functions. Consider this
question-and-answer response:

> (Q) What causes the fever to go up?
> (A) The attempt of the lymph in its circulation to adjust itself, or to
> destroy the infection through the liver and the spleen condition.
>
> 2456-4

The eighteen-year-old young man to whom the above excerpt was
directed had been diagnosed with acute lymphatic leukemia and was
"under the care of the best doctors at Mt. Sinai Hospital [in New York
City], who have treated his spleen with X-ray and given him several
transfusions," according to a letter from neurologist Dr. Fenton Taylor,
dated February 25, 1941. (2456-1, R-2) Between February 22 and May 8,
1941, he received six readings, several of which were quite brief and to
the point. His twin sister, who was present for the last two readings, was
very enthusiastic about them and insisted on their parents following
the suggestions. According to a notation made by Gladys Davis Turner
after speaking with the sister:

> . . . his mother is so overcome with the hopelessness of the condition,

she doesn't want to insist on him eating or drinking anything he doesn't want to [he couldn't handle liver as recommended in his diet, the orange juice hurt his throat, and the Atomidine placed in water gagged him]. The father is not "sold" on the readings—keeps saying that the doctors say it is not infectious because it can't be transmitted; that they've taken out the spleen and looked at it and it is all right. So, it seems very doubtful that the reading will be followed . . . Dr. William Taylor [an osteopath], present at the reading, told them they had everything to gain and nothing to lose by [following the reading].   2456-5, R-1

In his last reading, a reminder was given, perhaps also for his parents' benefit, of the proper motive and attitude that could in turn affect lymph flow:

. . . there should not be the attempts to aggravate but the attempt to get that reaction in the mental attitude of the *desire* of the body for purposeful activity. This will aid in the reaction of the lymph through the sympathetic nerve forces of the body, as much as all the doses that may ever be given.   2456-6

Problems with the spleen, a lymphatic organ, were addressed early on in his second reading:

As we find, the condition is primarily a glandular activity; an excess of destructive forces in the lymph as active by infection through the spleen—that has become somewhat engorged, and will gradually increase unless measures are taken.   2456-2

When asked what was the cause of the infection, the reading gave this reply:

. . . this began with an unbalancing of the glandular forces from lack of iodine in system. This then, with the unbalance, caused an infection in spleen and the gland that assimilates this in its refraction is causing in the lymph that dryness, hardness, as will be found indicated along the rib area of the body—or spine.   2456-2

As alluded to earlier, [2456] could not tolerate some of the recommended treatments, so questions were asked regarding this difficulty; for example, suggestions for various ways to prepare liver to make it more palatable to his taste (cooking suggestions that many of us might also find valuable and helpful!). The sister, however, was evidently unable to fully persuade the parents to follow through wholeheartedly, and a letter dated July 22, 1941, mentioned that the writer had "heard in some indirect way that [2456] died, but I do not know this on any real authority." No further verification is made of this possibility or of [2456]'s outcome.

Another person, a sixty-year-old woman, asked in her second reading on August 28, 1935, about her fluctuating temperature:

> (Q) What has been causing the slight temperature, and now subnormal?
> (A) The indications, as we have given, of the inflammation in the areas indicated. With the relaxing of the body, the subnormal temperature arises from too great a flow of the lymph to cleanse the portions of the body. Hence the applications of those things suggested.   882-2

Early on, the reading mentioned "a congestion in the functioning of the organs; especially kidneys and bladder" that was causing the inflammation. Deficiencies in the blood supply and disturbances in the nervous system were creating fatigue and exhaustion. The section of the reading describing her difficulties concluded, "Hence the local conditions are produced that bring about great distresses for the body."

Suggestions to alleviate these distresses included a series of massages "osteopathically given" with emphasis on her lumbar and coccyx areas; a formula, consisting of heated mutton suet, spirits of turpentine, spirits of camphor, and compound tincture of benzoin, to be administered in the evening across the lower back and kidney area; hot salt packs; colonics; and dietary advice, "an outline" of foods to be consumed at the morning, noon, and evening meals.

The reading also noted digestive problems: "the body responding at times very erratically to various foods or properties taken." Mention was made that certain types of food—certain kinds of milk, cheese, fruit (peaches and grapes)—"will not digest properly with the flow of the gastric forces in the system. Hence this has been or is a primary condition." (882-2)

Earlier, she was told by Cayce that "there has been a depletion in the red blood cells, there has also been a depletion in the lymph or the white blood or the warrior cells; so that the coagulation being bad makes for used energies with congestion, producing areas where a great deal of pain is at times experienced." (882-2)

In a letter written six days before her second reading (her first was a life reading), she described her physical condition:

> For two weeks I have been running a slight temperature due to an infection which has shown up in blood, pus, and albumin in urinalysis. The blood has cleared up but the last analysis still showed pus and the temperature persists. I don't want to go to a hospital for exploratory work, for it is not only expensive but most painful and a shock to the system which retards recovery.
>
> I am much underweight and Dr. Waters [Lulu Irene Waters Hare, D.O.], who has been treating me, thought the treatments, diet, and vibratory treatments would clear up the trouble. She is not satisfied with what she has accomplished, so wanted me to write you to locate the seat of the infection and tell what treatment to pursue to clear it up. Also what foods are best to increase my weight and build up my resistance.
>
> I have not been able to take liquids (milk, etc.) on account of gas and cannot take care of fats and sweets.
>
> Other than some irritation at times, I have had no pain. Do have occasional headaches.
>
> The trouble has seemed in the neck of the bladder, *but* we don't know.
>
> I shall be at home all Friday and Saturday resting and shall be very quiet on those days at 11:00 a.m. and 3:00 p.m. when I know you usually read. Hope you can give me an answer by Monday morning when I go to Dr. Waters again.   882-2, B-1

Twelve days after her reading, she wrote that Dr. Waters had been following the instructions in treating her and added, "The temperature started again just after I wrote you and I still have it . . . The reading spoke of pains, but I have no pains nor have I had any. Am hoping that the fever will soon clear up and that I shall have a little more pep." (882–2, R–1)

Four weeks later, Dr. Waters replied to a mailed questionnaire that [882] "was running a temperature of 99.6, sometimes a little less and sometimes more every day. There was considerable blood, also pus in the urine." She then listed a number of other observations, including "pain in right arm and shoulder." She ended her report by noting that her osteopathic diagnosis did not agree with the reading's, as she had "found much trouble in the cervical and upper dorsal area." (882–2, R–3)

On December 28, 1935, Mrs. [882] wrote, "I am very much better, but have not yet been able to gain any flesh." (882–2, R–5) Her son and her husband, who had also received readings and had been cause for much of her anxiety, were also doing well. No further information exists.

A fourteen–year–old girl, suffering from epilepsy, asked this in her second reading: "Why do no attacks occur when there is fever in the body?" Before answering, the Cayce source wanted to emphasize his accuracy! Here is the complete reply:

> This should be an indication to those who would study such conditions that the information coming through this channel knows what it's talking about! For the fever makes for an increase in the flow of the lymph through the body. Hence all those areas where there are the adhesions and those portions that are attempting to be broken up, these then contract with the cold or the less high temperature in the body, see? As these are gradually broken up, we will find there will be less and less of the attacks.   728-2

In this instance fever—as heat—increases lymph flow as well as helps break up adhesions. In another reading this caution was given: "Do not allow the body to be burned with the fever to the extent that the lymph becomes deadened. Massage, after the reduction, with equal parts of olive oil and tincture of myrrh, over the whole of the lymphatic circulation especcially, and along the center in the spine." (852–1) The fever was to be reduced by alcohol rubs, a common method for fever reduction, along the spine and at the base of the brain.

TUMORS, CYSTS, LUMPS, KNOTS, GROWTHS

While definitions of these items—tumor, cyst, lump, knot, growth—may overlap, there is usually no mistaking their appearance or the heightened concern over their appearance. Their sudden discovery in certain strategic body areas may trigger alarm bells, panic, apprehension, or perhaps a soothing denial of their potential danger. Their relationship to the lymph system constitutes, according to the Cayce readings, an important element in body functioning, offering what appears to be a unique perspective on this as-yet little understood or recognized component of the physical body. The Cayce viewpoint, as noted in earlier chapters, will be presented here with corresponding extracts and information, but first a few definitions.

A *tumor* refers to a swelling or new growth of tissue generally characterized by uncontrolled, progressive cell multiplication. The growth is considered faster than normal, creating a mass of abnormal tissue, either benign or malignant, that has formed and arisen from the cells of preexistent tissue. It appears to arise without cause and has no physiologic use or function.

With a somewhat different distinction, a *cyst* is an abnormal sac or capsule that contains a semisolid material, a liquid, or a gas. It has usually a thick membrane lined with epithelium cells that enclose the substance or material in a type of pocket. Though most are harmless, cysts may become malignant.

Any abnormal swelling or solid mass of an indefinite shape or size is considered a *lump.* Lumps can be formed by tumors or cysts or they can arise as a type of swelling or protuberance after a sharp blow or strike to the area.

Knots are any knoblike swellings or protuberances, usually firm or hard to the touch, such as a knot in a muscle. These lumps appear in or on a body part, a bone, or a body process.

Anything that grows can be called a *growth,* so by definition can include any abnormal mass or proliferation of tissue, such as a tumor. It can also refer to any abnormal formation of such matter or tissue that develops in or on the body.

In a similar category of abnormal growth, an additional term used frequently in the Cayce readings is **pockets,** such as "lymph pockets." A pocket, of course, can mean any small bag or pouch that holds something, a cavity or sac or enclosure that contains something. This descriptive term from the readings conveys the meaning of specific formations as a result of collections of lymph fluid, usually from poorly circulating or stagnant lymph flow. Excluding this latter definition of terms, none of the preceding items mentions lymph either in its formation or composition. Yet, regardless of this oversight, those individuals who presented their concerns to Cayce had just as much fear or worry about these growths in their bodies and wondered what to do about them as their present-day contemporaries.

Here is a sampling of extracts designating the role of lymph in the formation of these abnormalities:

One woman, told that she had "[l]ymph tumor tendencies," was suffering the effects of cold and congestion "and the weakened condition especially through the lymph in the assimilating system . . . " A reduction in her white blood supply resulted from her body trying to supply energies to her system. "And this has so thinned the walls as to cause soreness in portions of the lymph flow"—in the gall duct area, the pancreas, around the kidneys, and the organs of the pelvis—"all suffer as of a drying; thus reducing the supply to superficial circulation." Depending upon her ability "to cause better conditions in this assimilation as to bring about greater strength to the body," she might or might not develop "nodules or puffy conditions in lymph pockets" throughout her body. Tendencies toward lymph tumors could be corrected by stimulating the superficial circulation, getting osteopathic adjustments "to cause better distribution of eliminations," and following a better diet. "Do these things and we will have better results," the reading (2085-5) promised.

In another reading, [2863] was told that inflammation was in her ovary as well as in the alimentary canal, and phlegm was present at times in her teeth, gums, and throat areas, even in her stool. She asked, "Is there any tumor or growth anywhere?" The answer: "Rather the accumulation of lymph that forms and then disintegrates . . . If these accumulations form and remain, and then harden, they would be tumorous." (2863-2)

Another woman asked about her allergic reactions—"intense pain and pressure over the eyes lasting for days at a time"—when she came into contact with smoke, dust, and certain foods and plants. These could be relieved, the reading stated, by gentle massages plus a change in her mental attitude. The reading concluded: "For we see the sources of this are the incoordination between the superficial—or the lymph—and the deeper circulation, tending to form lymph tumors through the body." (3040-1) "Superficial" is the opposite of "deep," so what is referred to as "superficial circulation" is usually that area just under the skin surface, where—it is estimated—40-80 percent of the body's lymph vessels lie. Perhaps this explains why a number of readings (such as 2085-5, quoted earlier) recommended stimulating the superficial circulation as part of one's corrective regimen.

Other reasons for tumor formation involve the physical body becoming unbalanced chemically in a number of ways: "through congestion, through the non-elimination of poisons, through the non-emptying of those various portions where there are the tendencies to form lymph pockets, these might become tumorous—or might even become of a more serious nature . . . " (2581-1)

Another indication for the formation of a tumor was addressed in this young man's reading:

> (Q) What is the nature of the tumor on right knee cap?
> (A) Only that of the skin reaction, or the activity of the capillaries or lymph forming in the system, showing proper drainage is not taking place and eliminations not carried on properly.   2682-3

This twenty-three-year-old man had several months earlier been operated on for "a sort of flesh and blood clot—or tumor—which came from a blow given him by a baseball when he was just a youngster. He has had it for years and years and it has grown very large," reported his sister in a letter to Edgar Cayce (2682-1, B-1). The mass of tissue in his right groin was removed, but he experienced complications resulting from an infection following the surgery and eventually spent a month at the Cayce Hospital in Virginia Beach recuperating. "I am lost for words, to explain all the good it [Cayce Hospital stay] has done for me," he wrote in a letter to Gladys Davis on January 27, 1930, three days before his birthday (2682–4, R–1). Naturally, with all the serious difficulties he had experienced with the surgery, he was concerned about the appearance of a tumor on his right kneecap. Being told it was from a "skin reaction," lacking proper drainage, in which the lymph vessels were unable to transport excess fluid, and because of "eliminations not carried on properly," he asked immediately if a tumor is apt to return to his right side or any other body part in the future and was reassuringly told, "No."

Another man's inhaling of particles into his lungs eventually caused a lymph tumor to form as his body tried to fight against it (2685–1). In a number of cases, the readings mentioned that the body's attempts to right itself, to throw off toxins, to fight foreign particles result in "accumulations of the lymph pockets that produce the tumors . . . " (2945–1) Similarly, one woman was told: " . . . if there were to become accumulations in lymph pockets, in the soft tissue of the abdomen or in other portions of the body, these might cause tumors." (3291–1)

Another woman asked about and was given the exact location of her tumors:

> (Q) How many fibroid tumors have I on uterus and where are they, inside or outside?
> (A) At the mouth there are two. On the outside there is one. *None inside.*
> These are *not* fibroid; they are, as indicated more of the lymph accumulation; for fibroid becomes centralized or there is an affixation with which there gathers those of the nature that gradually builds to same. *This,* as you find, makes for a giving and then expanding again, or a rising and falling, owing to the irritations or owing to the general activity.   1140-2

The characteristic "rising and falling," or the forming and disintegrating of the accumulations of lymph, is spoken of in a slightly different way in another reading, this one in reference to [257]'s colon. While the above extracts mentioned tumors, the following referred to the formation of cysts:

(Q) Is the body forming new pockets in colon, or am I overcoming same? (A) We do not find new pockets that are not of a normal nature. Remember—as indicated time and again—these pockets are oft the attempt of the system, through the lymph pocket, to discharge those influences that act as assimilating things. These form and then discharge, but this is not of the nature that is detrimental unless they form and *do not* discharge—as was the case with that removed, see? [He had earlier had surgery to remove intestinal polyps.] These form and do not discharge, by those formations in the system from conditions where coagulation is produced that prevents lymph from being discharged. While there must be perfect coagulation in the internal as well as lymph flow and the like, these *can* or do at times—in bodies where there are the tendencies for accumulations—form pockets that become either adherences or gristly portions, or cysts, or conditions in the lymph itself such that there may be pockets in muscle, in tissue, in groin, in any portion where there are quantities of lymph flow—so that *through* the adherence such conditions are caused at times. These in themselves may become such as to produce protuberances or formations that may grow and then disintegrate.   257-238

We are perhaps more familiar with the term *coagulation* in reference to blood clotting, for example, when the blood changes from a fluid state to a thickened mass in order to seal an open wound and prevent further blood loss or hemorrhaging. Along these same lines, however, a clumping, thickening, or congealing can occur in other areas of the body, disturbing the free flow of lymph—slowing it down or hindering its flow in some way, as described in the above reading. For a woman, [817], who was experiencing a slowdown of circulation in her kidneys and bladder, what was needed, her reading explained, were certain additional elements

... that may be assimilated by the body to make not only solvents for the crystallizations that occur in the form of accumulations in cysts in portions of the lymph and in the soft tissue in parts of the body at times, where they tend to separate for themselves or the system attempts to produce coagulation around same to throw them off from the system,

but to make for the creating of that proper balance in the activity of the
organs themselves.   817-1

This adult female (no age recorded) had only one reading, which was
given on February 7, 1935, in Washington, D.C. Cystitis, her main complaint, is an inflammation of the bladder resulting from an infection
coming from either the urethra or the kidneys. The elements to "be
added in the physical and material manner," as her reading stated, included use of the Wet-Cell Battery, an herbal tonic, massages, as well as
beef juice and raw, fresh vegetables. She was also advised to seek the
services of a neuropathic physician. The reading concluded with this
reminder about the effect of attitudes upon the physical body:

> Keep that attitude which should be commendatory to every individual,
> for while physical forces are disturbed and while the mental attitude
> keeps for the body that which is of creative energy in itself, the *body* is
> built of that it assimilates; necessitating, then, the removal of pressures
> that have caused disturbance in this assimilation, and the addition of
> those properties as indicated for creating the proper balance. 817-1

Surgery to remove a lymph cyst was advised in Mrs. [2089]'s second
reading, because "from its formation [it] has begun to gather those forces
from the glandular activity of the system, and thus necessitates removal;
else it would cause a greater disturbance and faster growth." When asked
if the growth was "of a sarcoma nature," she was told it was not—at least
"in the present"—but it was "a lymph cyst—with a center that might
become anything!" However, preparations for surgery were to take into
account better coagulation: "there should *not* be the operation until the
test of the blood shows sufficient of the element to cause proper coagulation." (2089-2)

She also asked about what treatments she should follow after the
operation and was told to rest and to use the Wet-Cell Appliance plus
"all forms of creative influences of [a] suggestive nature," meaning positive, repetitive affirmations, use of reveries, or perhaps some hypno-
therapy.

What is interesting here is that this forty-four-year-old woman had already had surgery one month ago. Her first reading, done ten days later while she was still in the hospital, gave these simple instructions for recuperation: "The only suggestions we would make would be for a more hopeful, helpful and creative outlook or attitude." (2089-1) After six to eight weeks she could request another reading for more detailed suggestions.

A letter to her mother–in–law (who asked for the reading) from Hugh Lynn Cayce was enclosed with her first reading and contained this advice, also perhaps explaining the brevity of the reading:

> Evidently, it would be unwise to interfere with any of the recuperative treatments that are being given in the hospital at this time. Just as soon as she goes home from the hospital, please advise us and we will make another appointment for a reading—as is indicated in this information would be advisable. I'm sure that then we will be able to secure a complete analysis of her condition and suggestions for treatments. At this time it would be difficult to get any treatments carried out in the hospital that might be suggested.
>
> Of course, there would be no charge—further charge on your membership—for such an additional reading.   2089-1, R-1

Yet, during the operation, which involved attaching her intestine to her stomach, the surgeon discovered a large swelling the size of an orange and chose not to remove it because of the possibility of hemorrhage. So a follow–up reading was anxiously sought, being given the next day. According to the information already presented above, when her body was prepared and ready, she would need a second surgery to remove the lymph cyst. Unfortunately, no documentation exists as to the outcome.

A notation placed in brackets was made in another woman's reading (no age mentioned). Given on March 4, 1933, reading 292–1 contained this question: "Is there any lump in the right breast?" and in brackets following it were placed, followed by a question mark, the words "Lymph cyst?" Sometimes to help explain further or clarify certain terms from the Cayce source, Gladys Davis would add, enclosed in brackets, phrases or words that she thought would aid the one receiving the reading. Or they might have been inserted at a later date as questions would arise about certain terms or phrases. Because she had heard so many of the readings, taking them down in shorthand and typing them out to mail to the receiver, she developed a knack for interpreting the information or making it more meaningful and understandable. Perhaps this was why she added the questionable words: lymph cyst. Actually, in two later readings—not in earlier ones—the term "lymph cyst" was used, but as it was rather infrequent—and coming at a later date!— we can only speculate as to the reason this addition was inserted. It might, of course, have been written in at a later date. Yet here is the answer to [292]'s question:

> As we find, there has been a tendency for the glands that come to those activities over or under the right arm to be carrying more of those fluids than necessary; but with those activities that come from a stimulation to those of the exterior circulation, or to that called the superficial activity of the glands and their stimulation to the mammary glands, will remove any disturbance in this portion of the body; for the relaxations that will be received through those physical activities as given (not too strenuous, but those that make for the coordinating of the impulses from the centers along the spine) will bring about normalcy in these directions.
>
> 292-1

Her system had been experiencing difficulties with assimilation, the reading stated, and advised a series of "systematic" exercises along with baths and "rubs" (massages). After two to three weeks of such activities, she was to rest for two to three weeks. This series may have been what the reading excerpt referred to as "physical activities," which was predicted would "bring about normalcy" in her condition. This was her only reading; no documentation exists, so we do not know the results.

Lymph pockets, as noted earlier, appear to come and go, depending upon the reactions in one's body. In other words, certain physiological conditions can create these pockets, and when the individual would follow specific recommendations, the condition could also reverse itself; that is, the lymph pocket could be absorbed back into the body. For one woman, "the non–activity of eliminations" created the pockets, causing pressures in the body's internal system and "making for a drying effect or a slowed circulation through the sympathetics . . . " She asked whether the lump in her throat was related to her thyroid or was it "lymphatic," and the reading said it was the latter. It arose "from those tendencies for stoppages in portions of the circulation due to the at-tempts of the system to make for a *balancing* in a condition that needs attention . . . in the liver, gall duct area, the pancreas and the spleen . . . " (1140-1) With the proper stimulation, drainage of the area, osteopathic manipulations, and a diet "for a building up of the system," the condi-tions would clear up. Even the fibroid tumors in and around her uterus, which the reading said were "rather the pressures upon the organs by the improper drainages because of the disturbings in the circulation," could be absorbed provided "the proper drainages [be] set up . . . " This condition, of course, would be better than surgery. Then the reading stated:

> But the system itself, properly balanced, takes care of excesses even; though necessarily slower than operative forces, but safer—without those choices for the reaction from scar tissues' effect or the accumu-lation of lymph pockets or of irritations that make for fibrous reaction.
>
> 1140-1

Allowing the balanced physical body to do its thing was better than surgical procedures ("operative forces"), in which scar tissue, lymph pockets, or other irritations could occur as a result. Even the largest tumor in her uterus, one that was the size "of a wren's egg," which the reading called a lymph sac, could be absorbed.

Two instances in which "knots" were mentioned in the description of a person's physical status involved poor coordination. In the first, 2148-5, the receiver was a young boy whose first reading was given at two months and his last (number seven) at two years. He had been strug-gling with a fever, with "cold and congestion," so much so that the read-ing described it as "disturbing conditions . . . arising from old disturbances . . . " This affected the activity of his liver, pancreas, spleen, and kidneys as well as upsetting his lymph circulation "and has pro-duced those kernels or knots in various portions of the body. They may be indicated under the skin, in the neck, in the groin, under the arm, around the throat and the like," some of the principal areas where lymph nodes are present. To break up the lesions which had begun to form along the cerebrospinal system, this two–year–old was to receive three or four osteopathic adjustments "about a week apart," have a gentle massage before bedtime, drink a mineral compound in the mornings, and follow specific dietary suggestions. Two weeks after the reading, on February 5, 1942, his mother wrote: "We can't ever finish thanking you for giving us the readings. [His parents and aunt also received readings.] They did a world of good. [2148] is getting so big . . . He is looking much better, thanks to you." (2148–5, R–1)

The second instance mentioning knots was for a woman whose reading described "a heaviness almost as neuralgia, through the muscular forces in the back." (Neuralgia is pain along the course of a nerve.) Because of this poor coordination, lymph began to accumulate, forming knots "or the gatherings of lymph pockets." (5127–1) Lymph, which starts out fluid and watery, evidently can thicken, become sluggish, and eventually accumulate or come to rest in pockets, gradually forming tougher and harder knots or growths.

One reading noted that "accumulations from the lymph . . . may either be absorbed through the system or they may be removed [by surgery] as they separate themselves in the system," presumably by hardening and forming tumors that interfere too much "with the general circulation." (587–2) The possibility of the pockets becoming harder, interfering with or obstructing the circulation, was a process to be mindful of, potentially necessitating their removal through surgery.

Imagine someone's relief when asking, as Mrs. [690] did, "Is this a cancerous growth?" and receiving this answer: "Not a cancerous growth. Only lymph." (690–1) In addition to a weight problem, which was affecting her liver, she was also experiencing

conditions in the organs of elimination that prevent the proper drainages or proper eliminations of poisons. These tend to make for an accumulation in the lymph circulation, so that in the glands and in the soft tissue—as the abdominal area, as through the mammary glands—we have an accumulation of excess. These, as we find, are produced by

disturbing conditions in that gland [liver?] which both secretes and
excretes for the system.   690-1

She was also experiencing a "singing in the ear at times," burning
eyelids, bad taste in her mouth, and difficulty with eliminations just
before her menstrual period. Eventually, the kidneys were affected, but
it was not uremic poisoning. Unless corrected, her reading stated,

> there will be the production of the lymph ducts becoming involved to
> such an extent as to produce engorgements or growths . . . especially
> the ducts in the bile duct area, as to cause greater distresses. 690-1

Improper elimination and poor hepatic circulation produced these
irritations.

When unbalanced, irritating conditions exist, such as heightened
acidity in one's system—as was the case with Mrs. [805], which caused a
slowdown in her eliminations in the jejunum and in the alimentary
canal—lymph circulation, in turn, becomes sluggish; for Mrs. [805], it
caused the slowing of her peristaltic action.

> (Q) Have I any internal growth?
> (A) No. Not as such. There are natural inclinations where there is the lack
> of the lymph and emunctory activity through the torso of the system, by
> the clearing of the activities in the system, to form—as it were—in groups;
> that become at times lymph pockets, but these have not segregated or
> formed themselves into growths.   805-3

To bring reactions back to a near normal state, she was advised to
take Ventriculin to stimulate gastric flow, but if this was not sufficient,
she could give herself enemas with baking soda and, at the last rinse,
Glyco-Thymoline; these alkaline properties would "*gradually* aid the colon itself to absorb and build that necessary activity from such an influence."

One fifty-five-year-old woman, who received a total of forty-two
readings from 1929 to 1943, had a check reading on tumor tendencies,
as she had previously had surgery to remove some knotty tumors from

her spine and leg. She asked, "Have the growths that were in my lymph circulation been eliminated?" "Not entirely," the answer came, "else there would be better lymph flow through the body." (303–32) She was advised to "keep very close" to the recommended treatments, which included steams, massages, osteopathy, enemas, and certain vitamins.

What other effects can result from lymph pockets? According to this reading, one cause may produce a variety of effects:

> At other periods we will find that from the very same cause there will be a different complication, when certain characters of foods or activities of the body will affect the lymph flow through the trunk portion of the system. Or, through the upper digestive area we find the lymph pockets, as it were; causing gas pressures in the abdominal area, even a little nausea at times; and distresses to portions of the system as to affect even the locomotion.   1901-2

Earlier, this reading mentioned a "complication of disturbances" that could affect one's body and that "[t]hese affectations are in the lymph circulation . . . " The next chapter will discuss remedial applications suggested in the readings to assist lymph circulation.

Additional information on tumors.   The above section focuses on one aspect of the Cayce readings' information on lymph. Yet this material presents a unique view of the workings of the lymphatic system: the process by which tumors (or cysts, growths, and so forth) are created involves in a very direct way the flow or nonflow of lymph fluid. A number of readings describe in a consistent way the origin, formation, and development of tumors—if only in a brief sentence or two. To summarize, the scenario might be described as unfolding in this manner:

The fluid moving through vessels collecting hormones, proteins, and cellular waste products begins to slow down in some body areas. This stagnation may be due to inactivity or lack of movement, a buildup of toxins or increased acidity in the bloodstream, vertebral misalignments or subluxations in the spine, a dis-eased organ such as the liver or kidney, or several of these conditions all occurring in close time proximity to one another.

One person actually asked in his reading: "What causes the sluggish-

ness in the superficial lymph glands?" and note the emphasis given to
the importance of lymph coordination in his answer:

> That activity . . . in the non-functioning or over-coordination or over-
> balancing in those functionings of the glands . . . that make for their
> warring one with another in portions of the system. And these produce
> to the superficial circulation that lack of the sufficient energies to carry
> to the lymph circulation those influences necessary.
>
> O that there were more, as this body, who would consider that
> necessary coordination of the lymph and emunctory activities with
> those of the general circulation!
>
> Study it well in thyself, and thou wilt be able to give to others much
> that will add to the human hope in this experience!   1063-1

The reading was given on November 23, 1935, a time when so little
was known or understood about this function. We can speculate, perhaps, that the admonition to study and understand the function of the
lymph applies equally as well to present–day, health–conscious students
and interested individuals who may have identical questions and concerns as Mr. [1063]. To continue the scenario on tumor formation:

The unit that is our body begins to react to these unbalanced, unhealthy conditions, sending out signals of distress to aid the ailing parts.
Increased congestion and buildup of fluid may result from this effort to
heal. Symptoms now become recognized by the alert mind: achiness,
fatigue, congestion, sensory disturbances (changes in vision, taste, or
hearing), some painful areas—clues that something in our bodies is out
of kilter.

Now that we have definable symptoms, we can search our pharma-
copeia to decide what to do about them. The people who came to Cayce
seeking such advice had very often already contacted a medical doctor;
some were going through a series of remedies or had already completed the required, necessary treatments or surgeries; the medicines
they were prescribed to consume had already been taken. Yet some
chose to go a different route by contacting a psychic and see what further information and help they could obtain for their ailment. Often
their subsequent reading, then, mentioned a problem in the lymph sys-

tem along with other indications, or reference to it was made in response to specific questions submitted with the reading. In these instances remarks on the quality of lymph flow were noted along with
the progression of events causing it. While the next chapter will cover
the remedial suggestions, here we will present further information on
the causal formation of tumors.

To one woman this description was offered:

> . . . we find where glands become clogged by any secretion, or any
> condition in a system wherein cell tissue becomes broken, these lodge
> and form a condition that is set around by the leucocytes in the system,
> to attempt to prevent inroads in such tissue. In this condition here . . .
> we find tissue in the gland wherein this has become separated, but *not*
> set in the nature of that as is in the case of cells becoming cell building
> inside of the condition, see? for each cell of any nature, whether of the
> live tissue, in health or in disease, builds by separating . . . Hence the
> necessity . . . of the eliminations throughout the system being kept in
> an accentuated, yet not aggravated, condition, else, by creating aggra-
> vation in tissue, or in lymph, or in blood, there may be this same
> condition set up in other portions of the body. Not that the condition in
> itself is of the malignant nature as yet, for this is as of one separated only
> in the system of broken or of dead tissue *not* eliminated in the normal
> way and manner.   569-9

One of the proper functions of lymph is to transport dead, useless
cells to the body's eliminatory organs. Perhaps in [569]'s system, this
particular function was hindered. The reading was given on August 13,
1926. In a much later reading, on January 12, 1943, Miss [569] asked,

> (Q) What has caused this condition, and has it become a tumor?
> (A) An accumulation of poisons from general conditions . . . and it has
> formed into a lymph tumor. That it may become of a nature, or has
> formed into a nature already as to set up an activity within itself, is also
> indicated . . .   569-27

Because the lymph tumor was now in a better–formed, independent state—not dependent still on underlying tissue—Miss [569] could decide on her own, the reading stated, whether or not to have surgery to remove the tumor. Conditions were serious, and the surgery would alleviate, but not cure. In April 1943 Miss [569] received her final reading; according to a notation inserted by Gladys Davis within reading 569-9 (excerpted earlier), Miss [569] died in October 1943, following an operation to remove a cancerous tumor on her Fallopian tube.

One final note on tumor formation comes from [943], a forty-year-old man who received this reading on January 21, 1932. In response to a question on the cause and cure for psoriasis, he was given this information:

> As is known, psoriasis is—itself—an infectious condition that affects the emunctory and lymph circulation, and causes an improper coordination of the eliminating forces of the system, as in this body. Would this not be thrown off in the epidermis, or the lymph and capillary circulation, with this particular condition of this body, the intestinal tract would be full of pinholes; or, were it to go to the lungs, there would be tuberculosis; were it to go to the valves of the heart, it would be heart trouble—as would be called; were it to go to the liver, it would be cirrhosis of the liver; were it to go to the spleen, it would be a hardening of one end of it; were it to go to the brain, it would be softening of the brain; were it to go to the glands of the throat or thyroids, it would be that of goiter; or were it to settle in some other portion—were it to *settle*—it would become a tumor of some character or nature.   943-17

Though these possibilities may relate to this particular person, yet the excerpt is interesting in explaining how anyone's body might deal with "infectious" forces.

When a tumor becomes malignant.   What tips the scales from benign to malignancy? This question is of the utmost concern for those who know of or have discovered a growth somewhere in their bodies but don't have as yet an accurate diagnosis or verdict as to its status. What eventually determines the major change from a safe—hence benign—tumor to one that is destructive and potentially life-threatening? A number of excerpts from the Cayce readings describe this condition:

how tumors may become malignant. One reading states:

> ... when cellular forces become so aggravated, either by bruising or lack
> of elements in the system to keep a continuity of life force, they set up
> within themselves. Thus they draw upon the system, becoming—
> *ordinarily,* and oftentimes—malignant in their nature.   1013-1

What kind of bruising in the cells would create such a disturbance?
What could interrupt the "continuity of life force" that would eventually begin to put a drag on or drain the system?

Several other readings mention irritations that could elicit changes
leading to a malignancy. One reading noted an "improper coagulation
through the blood and lymph forces" that would cause "adherences or
sticking, or the accumulations that form more in the lymph—though if
irritated they might become malignant." (2529-1) So here the lymph
itself seems to be the terrain where such a malignancy might occur.

Irritations are also mentioned in another reading in which stickiness
like an adhesive tape eventually creates adhesions and lesions, if certain former conditions appear. Here is the excerpt:

> ... there is the inclination for the activity of the lymph to produce pain
> or drawing in the manner as if one were pulling or removing an adhesive
> from a portion of the body . . .
>
> If there is the reverting to the conditions that cause superacidity,
> overaggravation by cold and congestion, we may produce greater
> adhesions, greater lesions; and eventually cause irritations that would
> become malignant in their nature . . .
>
> Hence the necessity for the *system's* being kept near normal to
> prevent it becoming a more serious condition.   1446-3

Note the strong influence and effect that acidity and congestion have
on one's system. Note also the words that seem to denote more of an
extreme situation—*superacidity, overaggravation, greater* adhesions and lesions—as if it is these exaggerated conditions that spell danger or trouble
for the body.

In another reading irritations in the bladder or the urethra may "become malignant" if precautions are not taken, one man was told. He had been under a lot of stress (financial, marital, and so on), which the reading acknowledged and strongly advised him to keep away from any intoxicants—beer, wine, *any* alcohol—as these would exacerbate his anxiety. He was warned: "Unless these precautions are taken, this will become deeper and deeper-seated. And . . . may produce such an irritation in the bladder, or such an irritation in the urethra, as to become malignant. Better take precautions *now!*" (391-17) In this case stress is a predominant indicator of a tendency toward malignancy.

The reminder that cancer cells are actually present in everyone was noted in one thirty-year-old man's reading when he asked if there were any symptoms of cancer in his system. After stating that there were not any symptoms of cancer, the reading continued: "Remember, for every individual physical body what might be sometimes called symptoms are ever present. But the breaking of cells, injury to some portions of the body, these are usually the sources and the activities that bring about such." (533-18) So again, the "breaking of cells" and injuries, possibly repetitive injuries, may be the source of malignancies or the trigger for such dangerous conditions to develop.

One woman who had "a complication of disturbances" that were described as "localized, working one against another; thus showing an incoordinating and an uncooperative influence working within the physical forces of the body," was told that a deep-seated catarrhal condition existed (1762-1). This congestion resulted in a thickening of tissue in her body's mucous membranes—throughout her digestive system, throat, bronchi, even her pelvic organs—forming "nobules in the lymph." While they were not cancerous, the reading said they "may become such if they are bruised or if there is a breaking of the cellular force . . . " (1762-1) What began in her system as an incoordination could lead to a malignancy if the cells became broken or bruised, similar information to what was mentioned in previous readings extracts.

What would cause the bruising or the breaking up of cells? Hard, strong knocks or blows—perhaps repeatedly to the same area—tears in muscles from strenuous exercise or a sports injury, deep pressure from massages that are applied with too strong back-and-forth gliding movements or rubbing too heavily across the tissue, severe overacidity in the bloodstream, poor or irregular eliminations, maybe even some surgical procedures are potential causes implicated in bruising or broken cells. These somewhat extreme conditions are perhaps what puts the body out of balance to such an extent that the irritations presented by lymph pockets or tumors may become malignant.

One forty-year-old man was told that his skin condition for which he was being treated was "now more or less of a malignant nature, though not what is ordinarily in some conditions called cancerous; but has been a sluffing of the portions of affectations by the very deadening of the affected area by the high vibratory forces produced from such strong X-Ray reactions and properties in system." (1242-6)

He had received a fuller explanation in an earlier answer when he asked about the nature of his skin condition. A disturbance in his scapula (shoulder blade), he was informed, eventually caused irritations in his neck and side of face. "And the application of the exceedingly high vibratory forces produced such a rate of change as to make for that nearer to a malignant nature. Thus the manner in which sluffing and deadening of portions of affected areas became as discharges and the conditions that produced the nature of that which has been part of the reaction." (1242-6) In both explanations the Cayce source used the phrase "high vibratory forces," which evidently increased the rate of cell changes, resulting in a malignancy but not necessarily a cancerous condition. Then Mr. [1242] asked:

(Q) What is the disease known as cancer?
(A) . . . there are many varied kinds of cancer. Nineteen—as we find—variations or formations, externally, internally, stony, and the variations that arise from glandular or organic disturbance, or infectious forces that arise from bruises or from all the various natures from which these come; each having a variation according to that portion of the system or its cycle in which the affectation takes place.   1242-6

Not only is bruising again mentioned as a cause, but the information noting the variety and types of cancer is also food for thought. This reading, by the way, was given in 1936.

When asking for advice—"either physical or spiritual"—[1242] was told:

There should be kept, to be sure, a hopeful, constructive attitude as to its material and physical welfare, as well as in its spiritual application and spiritual attitudes. For each soul should gain that understanding that whatever may be the experience, if there is not resentment, if there is not contention, if there is not the giving of offense, it is for then that soul's own understanding, and will build within the consciousness of the soul itself that which may bring the greater understanding of the spiritual in the physical body.

Then let the prayer, the meditation, ever be:

Here am I, Lord. Thou knowest my faults, Thou knowest my weaknesses: yet I am Thine, and Thou would use me as Thou seest fit. Let Thy will, O God, be done in and through me, in such measures that I may be a channel of blessings to others. For as I forgive, may I be forgiven. As I bless may I be blessed by Thy love and Thy presence.

Then keep me in the ways, in body, in mind, in spirit, that I should go.   1242-6

A hopeful, constructive attitude matched with prayer and meditation will provide the keys to a better consciousness, a better healthy state for one's entire being. Yet the physical body, as an entity, is a miracle world unto itself, capable of renewal and rejuvenation. From time to time the Cayce readings remind us of this wonderful system and the tremendous accomplishments of which it is capable. Here is one such excerpt acknowledging the body's activities. (Note that the lymph is here considered a component of the blood system, which, given its circulatory function, has a predominant role in rebuilding.)

Each portion of the body—as the sensory system; as the activity of lungs, heart, liver or kidneys, as well as digestion or assimilation and distribution of that assimilated—reproduces through the body from that assimilated not only the supplying forces for various functionings of the complex activities of the body, but rebuilds itself. The greater portion of this, to be sure, is carried on through the blood systems; that is, the lymph, the emunctory, as well as the flow of white and red blood corpuscles, as well as the leukocyte or that form in the lymph that aids in shielding or creating coagulation, or of putting over strained areas the

protective forces in the use of any portion of the body—whether it be the
muscular tendon or the activities in even the impulse of emotion or
body-force itself.   1770-6

The interrelationship of the many body parts reflects a oneness, a
unity, of the whole. It also represents a quality of the soul itself: coop–
eration. In the Search for God Study Group material, based on the 262
series of readings on soul development, cooperation is for seekers the
first step on the spiritual path. This aspect and principle is mirrored in
our physical bodies as well, with all the functions attempting to work in
harmony, assisting one another, and providing the needed activities of
renewal and protection for each to carry on its work. Thus is presented
to us a wonderful reflection and example of balance and harmony and life.

CONCLUSION

It may be easy to understand how lymph influences systemic condi–
tions in the physical body, given not only its pervasiveness but also its
relationship to the circulatory, digestive, and excretory systems. In presenting this information, certain characteristics of lymph emerged:
Lymph helps to aid or lubricate the whole bodily system, and when this
function is operating poorly, an imbalance arises in which too much
fluid occurs in one area and a drying effect occurs in another. Its role as
a digestive aid is demonstrated by the lacteals, present in the small
intestine, where the absorption of fat takes place. An additional role—as
a fighter of infection—is found in the Peyer's patches, also present in the
small intestine, which prevents bacteria from penetrating the intestinal
wall. Movement of lymph is necessary for proper peristaltic action
throughout the alimentary canal, and a poor or insufficient flow could
result in a fever. Fever also increases the flow of lymph. Accumulation
of lymph into "pockets" is the forerunner of tumors, cysts, and various
growths that may become hardened and eventually malignant. Infection, acidity, irritations, and congestion all affect lymph circulation.

The next chapter discusses various remedies from the Cayce readings
to help keep the lymph in a healthy, balanced state.

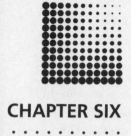

CHAPTER SIX

· · · · · · · · · ·

Applications for a Healthier Lymph

Those who are somewhat unfamiliar with the Cayce health readings may find the excerpts in the previous chapters difficult to read and comprehend. Probably those obtaining the readings did as well, considering their necessity at times for follow-up questions in subsequent check readings. If the recipients were working with a physician or other health care professional and presented their reading to this person, the medical provider seemed to grasp and understand to some extent the information being presented, as reflected in his or her responses to questionnaires mailed out for follow-up documentation. Gladys Davis, Edgar Cayce, and Hugh Lynn Cayce through their letters helped with the interpretations as well.

One of the most positive, serviceable aspects of a Cayce reading is the often detailed regimen of treatment outlined for the ill individual to follow in order to get well. From the excerpts already presented in the previous chapters, one can view the range of options offered to the seeker, a holistic plan of health to those desiring some relief from their sickness. This chapter outlines some of those remedies that the readings stated were specifically beneficial to the lymphatic system.

INTERNAL APPLICATIONS

Starting first with items that are ingested or taken internally, we note that two were mentioned more frequently than others: saffron tea and olive oil.

Before offering an explanation of the reason for their use, however, an important note to be added here concerns any remedy you might choose to take or treatment protocol you might decide to follow. The readings were given for individuals. Even though the ailment or disease might be almost identical from one person to another, the regimens that were outlined matched the particular individual who requested the information. Attempts to follow someone else's reading may not always be effective. Review the suggestions found near the beginning of chapter 1 offering you guidelines for following a health reading. *You should always consult a physician or other health care professional for any medical problem and before altering or adding any treatment to your protocol.* The content of this book is not intended for self-diagnosis or self-treatment but as useful information to be worked with and applied in conjunction with proper medical advice and guidance from your own "inner physician."

Another important reminder regarding the listing of Cayce remedies recommended for use and application: Presenting such an itemized list camouflages the fact that these products were not taken in isolation; they were often used in combination with other remedies, appliances, and treatments—sometimes done in cycles with rest periods factored in to aid the body to absorb the good effects of the "medicines" and to readjust itself. It would be helpful to keep this in mind when deciding to try some of the suggested remedies, as rarely is just one item considered in treating any ailment successfully. Studying more fully and carefully specific readings or a series of readings on a particular health concern may better help you to determine the suitable method or path you would choose to undertake.

Saffron tea. Known as Yellow or American Saffron, this herb is used primarily for its perspiration-inducing quality and, because it coats the stomach, as an aid to digestion. This latter property was noted in a number of readings, even at times pinpointing specific locations, for example: "This [tea] will be active especially upon the digestive forces, or will keep the correct activity in such as to cause a better flow of the lymph through the tissue of the lower digestion in the pylorus, in the upper portion of jejunum, and especially in the lacteal duct center." (3109–1)

Another quality of the tea was stated here: "It stimulates better strength through the activities of the lymph and emunctory circulation in the alimentary canal." (257–215) Mr. [257] was told not to take it "in a haphazard manner," but drink it "for two, three, four, five days a week, ten days," then leave off a few days and resume "until there is a better condition physically created throughout the alimentary canal." Usually a pinch of the tea was put into a teacup, then boiling water poured over it, letting it steep from fifteen to thirty minutes. Strain and drink it, making the tea fresh each time. It is readily available in most grocery and health food stores.

Olive oil. Recommended for both external and internal uses, olive oil was mentioned in more than one thousand readings. Though not always specified, pure olive oil, what we might call "(first) cold pressed" or "extra virgin," would be the type of oil to ingest or to use as a massage lotion. (In about ten readings an olive oil shampoo was also mentioned.)

Mr. [900] was advised to take, along with his Yellow Saffron tea (half a glass two to three times a day), one to two teaspoonfuls of pure olive oil. Taken daily, it would "act as a lubricant and as food value for the inflammation as has been created through the whole intestinal tract . . . " (900–197) Another man was told that the olive oil would "produce for the lymph of the digestive system that proper balance which supplies the activity for the peristaltic movement of the muscular forces throughout the intestinal tract." (294–156) One twenty-six-year-old gentleman, who had a total of nine readings, was suffering from memory lapses and "falling conditions." When he asked about olive oil, he was told: "Olive oil, so it does not become rancid in the system, taken in small enough doses to assimilate, is helpful to any intestinal disturbance . . . " (567–7)

Cod liver oil. A fifteen-year-old girl, whose mother requested the reading, asked about taking cod liver oil, a common medicinal supplement "inflicted" upon many children for generations. Rich in vitamins A and D, it is obtained, as its name suggests, from the liver of the cod fish and other related fishes. The reading gave it a positive endorsement: "Cod liver oil, of course, is an addition to a developing body in making for not only the structural activity, but throughout the lymph and all that necessary to supply the vitamins needed." (276-5) The brand recommended was White's Cod Liver Oil tablets; she was to take "two [tablets] after meals (only twice a day) . . . [for] periods of three to five days, then rest for periods of an equal length of time. But take sufficient to have the desired effect." The answer concluded with this statement: " . . . more *often* it will be found that the activity from what is known as the [homeopathic] doses is the better; even of [allopathic] medicine!" (276-5) Homeopathy, founded by Samuel Hahnemann (1755-1843), involves the administering of minute doses of a substance that is capable of producing symptoms of the disease being treated, hence its name, "homeo," meaning *like* or *similar*. (Allopathy is the opposite, involving treating the disease by producing conditions contrary or antagonistic to the illness.)

Cimex lectularius. One example of a homeopathic product is this rather unusual substance from a strange source. Cimex (pronounced "sigh-meks") lectularius, recommended about ten times in the readings, is made from bedbug juice (*cimex* is the scientific name, the genus, for bedbug). With a wry sense of humor, the Cayce source several times noted that its origin should perhaps be kept hidden from the recipient, as it "would not be very pleasant to the entity" (420-7), or "it might be offensive . . . " (1553-27) This remedy was recommended for cases of dropsy, an older designation for edema, or swelling, usually in the feet, ankles, and lower extremities, "caused by infiltration of the tissues with diluted lymph fluid." (*An Edgar Cayce Home Medicine Guide*, p. 27) Evidently, the Cimex lectularius would help relieve the condition as well as "control the lymph circulation . . . " (420-7) It can be purchased, no prescription needed, in health food stores that contain a homeopathy section.

Colonics. Sometimes called high enemas or colonic irrigations, these treatments also merit an "honorable mention" in the readings, owing to their frequent recommendation. As part of hydrotherapy, this internal cleansing helps stimulate the bowels, but it may also stimulate the kidneys. Warm, filtered water under pressure is gradually inserted into the large intestine, then allowed to flow out (release). This flushing action is repeated throughout the session, lasting nearly three-fourths of an hour. Given by a professional using a special machine, a colonic is noticeably different from an enema, as explained by Dr. Harold Reilly: " . . . an enema is a relieving process and a colonic is a stimulating and corrective process." (*The Edgar Cayce Handbook for Health Through Drugless Therapy*, p. 223) Enemas help clean and clear the lower bowel, or rectum, while a colonic, because of its extra pressure, helps cleanse the upper portion of the large intestine, removing more toxic material and stimulating the peristaltic action with its gentle water-massaging.

The readings also recommend solutions added to the water: a combination of baking soda and salt (a saline solution) to help with the releases, prevent irritation, and purify the lymph flow, and in the final rinses a dilution of Glyco-Thymoline, an alkalizing agent to the system as well as an intestinal antiseptic. (For more information on colonics, see *Edgar Cayce's Guide to Colon Care* by Sandra Duggan, R.N.)

A buildup of toxins in one's system can create a variety of symptoms, as noted from several of the cases mentioned in the previous chapters. One gentleman was told that unless better circulation was set up or proper lymph circulation was created, he would continue to have rashes. To achieve this stimulation of circulation, along with his other treatments, he was to have a colonic about every ten days until the circulation throughout his alimentary canal improved. (4079-1) One woman was advised to get colonics often, using the salt and soda combination, because they would "purify the movement of the activities of the lymph flow in the intestinal tract itself." (1010-21)

Coordination of various activities is noted as a priority in a number of health readings, implying a balance, or harmony, to be established among bodily systems. This man was told to have occasional colonics to cleanse his colon, but "do not take such oftener than once a month . . . " (2298-1) Using the solutions mentioned earlier, the colonic irrigation would not only tend to "cleanse the colon of the engorgement area, but to dilate and to supply activities direct that will coordinate with the lymph flow through the intestinal system." (2298–1)

The colonic, then, not only cleanses large wastes from the body but also opens pathways for the finer eliminations from lymph. As to whether or not one can benefit from or need such a treatment, consider this statement from the readings:

> Simply because there is an evacuation through the alimentary canal each day does not indicate at all times . . . that there is being a cleansing or a healthy condition throughout the intestinal tract. If this were true, we wouldn't have these pains, we wouldn't have these reactions!
>
> 567-7

This person suffered from painful intestinal gas, memory lapses, and epilepsy. In another reading, when asked about Epsom salts baths and colonics, Cayce gave this reply: "For, *every* one—everybody—should take an internal bath occasionally, as well as an external one. They would all be better off if they would!" (440–2)

Inhalant. This rather popular remedy, mentioned in more than three hundred readings, was recognized for its wide use in all sorts of respiratory problems. While the formula varied slightly in different readings, it usually contained pure grain alcohol to which was added a number of oils (eucalyptus, pine needles, rectified oil of turpentine) plus compound tincture of benzoin, tolu balsam, and rectified creosote. The solution, placed in a wide–mouthed jar, fills only a portion of the container; this is so that the fumes, after the bottle has been shaken, can be inhaled through a breathing tube placed in a hole in the lid. When not in use, corks are placed back into the holes. It is most effective when used regularly several times a day. One woman was given this information on its benefits:

> This will aid the sympathetic and the lymph circulation to alleviate irritations in the nasal passages and the head and antrum, as well as the throat and the bronchi and larynx, even the lungs themselves—for a stimulated circulatory force that would be most beneficial.   464-23

Another woman was told: "This is an antiseptic and a healer, and will prevent the sneezing, as well as the tendency for the lymph to drip from nostril and nasal passages." (2801-6) Today it is sold as Herbal Breathing™ by the official worldwide supplier of Cayce health care products.

Deep breathing.   Exercise was a big part of the Cayce protocol, but in this case breathing was emphasized along with it. One thirty-one-year-old woman was told to "massage the lymph centers—from the pubic center to the throat itself, and in the back of the neck, raising the head forward and the breathing brought into same—through the deep breathing." (3149-2) This massage area follows to some extent the position of the thoracic duct, the main lymphatic vessel in the body. The duct passes through the diaphragm (the diaphragmatic aortic opening), which upon deep breathing (both inhalation and exhalation), squeezes the lymph within it, forcing it to move and thus enhance circulation, allowing it to flow better throughout the body. In a follow-up question the information was repeated about massaging the lymph centers with this comment added: "You'll have to train this body almost how to breathe." (3149-2) Deep diaphragmatic breathing is now considered a necessary part of one's therapy for stimulating lymph circulation.

To end this section of the chapter, take note of this excerpt:

> . . . be mindful that all, in the way of *internal* medicine, is of the nature that is *allaying* to that of sore, ulceration, or stress; at the *same* time not subjugating same through that of hypnotics, or hypnosis, in a manner as to produce the greater strain, or the bleeding—whether through those of the lymph or those of the veins themselves . . .   5426-1

To "allay" means to bring relief or help to a painful or stressful condition. In making choices for our treatment remedies, we are reminded to consider their effects on our bodies. Presumably, we would be familiar enough—as much as possible—with our body's operation so as not to cause any undue stress and thus be able to determine wisely what we need for healing.

EXTERNAL APPLICATIONS

Not surprisingly, massages and spinal manipulations were most frequently noted for their effects on the lymphatic system. These remedies, mentioned consistently throughout the entire body of health readings, each had a special influence on lymph, especially concerning its eliminatory quality. Lymph, as a system, is often described as the body's garbage disposal network, collecting waste from the cells, shuffling toxins to the nodes to be filtered and purified, and helping the body excrete unwanted materials by transporting them to the appropriate eliminatory organs. In the Cayce readings' approach to health, the measures undertaken by the individual assist in the healing; they act as facilitators of the return to health. Though each remedy has its own particular brand or purpose or vibration for fostering healing, it does not in and of itself cause the healing. The readings are emphatic that healing comes from the Divine within each person, with the particular remedy aiding in the facilitation of that process.

Massage.   Considering that the skin is the largest organ as well as part of the elimination system, it is easy to understand how massage plays such an important role in assisting the lymphatics. Often the oils to be used were noted as well.

One woman was advised to have a massage over her joints and abdomen. The lubricant consisted of two ounces of olive oil, two ounces of peanut oil, and one-fourth of an ounce of liquefied lanolin. The skin would naturally absorb the oil, which would "act as a stimulating food value for the emunctory and lymph circulation . . . " (3337-1) Another woman, given the same combination of oils, was also told that it would stimulate lymph circulation (4054-1). In another reading a massage with peanut oil followed by an alcohol rub—using a mild solution of grain alcohol (not denatured or rubbing alcohol)—would "give strength and vitality to the tendons and muscles . . . give stimulating activity to the lymph and emunctory circulation of the abdomen *and* of the organs of same." (2642-1) One woman, unable to walk, was advised to get "massages of the limbs and the lower sacral and lumbar area, and abdomen . . . These will supply much of food value to the lymph and emunctory circulation through same." (3080-1) Following a hot bath, a massage with cocoa butter "in the areas where [osteopathic] corrections have been made" will supply "food for the lymph and emunctory circulation," another man was told. (3558-1)

To help dissolve an ovarian cyst, the reading for [3472] recommended placing Glyco-Thymoline packs over the groin area, followed by a "neuropathic massage, where the gland centers of the lymph circulation are stimulated to activity." She could also receive osteopathic treatments, if she so chose, but if the packs, massages, and adjustments were done, "we find that there may be the absorption of this cyst." (3472-1) A neuropathic massage is one that follows the nerve centers of the body. With the use of various massage strokes, circulation and flow of nerve impulses are improved. (See *Edgar Cayce's Massage, Hydrotherapy, and Healing Oils*, pp. 59-65, for a fuller description of a neuropathic massage.)

Cocoa butter was mentioned again as a beneficial lubricant for massage, and the effects on the skin were also described in this question and answer:

(Q) Would cocoa [butter] massage do this body good?
(A) The whole of the neuropathic massage would be well. This carries either cocoa or any of those properties that aid the skin or the epidermis to react to the stimulating effect given to the lymphatic or capillary circulation.   325-26

Olive oil and tincture of myrrh—equal portions—is a common massage lubricant in the readings. The oil is to be heated first, then the myrrh (which is an alcoholic solution) is added to the warm oil; this enables the two substances to blend better together and not to separate. Thus, it is to be made fresh with each massage treatment. One man was advised to have "a thorough massage . . . from the base of brain to the end of spine. Well that olive oil and myrrh be rubbed in near those portions of body where same will be absorbed or taken up by lymphatic circulation . . . " Later in the reading, these areas were pointed out: "Arm pits, across the abdomen, across the lower portion of the spine, and in the sides . . . " (4371-1) The skin's absorptive quality brings the healing oil right into the lymph vessels under the skin. In earlier readings quoted, note the references to the oil's value as a "food" for lymph.

Another man was given a regimen to be followed once a week: a Turkish bath (steam bath), followed by a salt rub, then a massage with a particular formula for the oil (one ounce of Nujol, one ounce of witch hazel, one ounce of olive oil, and one-half ounce of tincture of myrrh), ending with a grain alcohol rub. The reading then summarized:

> First the [bath with the] salt rub, then the application of this combination of oils for the eliminations and for the various portions of the lymphatic circulation, and then followed with the alcohol rub. This, as we see, will rid the system of these conditions in the joints, in and about the centers from the glands' secretion, and the whole general eliminations be kept nearer normal.   849-4

Nujol, an ingredient in the massage oil formula, is also called Russian White Oil, Usoline, or mineral oil and is suggested in a number of Cayce formulas that were prescribed for muscular sprains, strains, backaches, injured ligaments, and paralysis.

Spinal manipulation. Whether administered by an osteopath or a chiropractor, spinal manipulation is considered extremely beneficial, according to the readings, a number of which referred to its ability to establish equilibrium in the body. This characteristic was mentioned in the following excerpt as well as a further explanation of the purpose of manipulation: "to cause nature to produce a normal contraction of muscular forces and the nerve centers to function properly, to produce perfect equilibrium in distributing nerve energy to increase the circulation on the hepatics; the circulation between the liver and kidneys throughout the upper or negative poles, so that the lymphatics will carry nerve energy, and produce proper capillary circulation and elimination through the proper organs." (4137-1) Use of a remedy, such as manipulation, *as an aid* to better health is demonstrated clearly in this statement: helping the natural forces achieve results in the physical body.

Adjustments "make for the better flow of the lymph and the circulatory forces . . . " (567-8); they "assist the capillary and lymphatic circulation" (337-6). While these brief statements point out the connection that manipulations may establish between lymph and blood, another mentions the "coordination between the lymphatic and sympathetic nerve system and the cerebrospinal centers" that is created when the ganglia alongside the spine are stimulated. (2977-2) Ganglia are masses of nerve cells running parallel to the spine; they serve as centers from which nerve impulses are transmitted. These centers are stimulated, then, through spinal adjustments.

One man asked if later in life he would have a tendency toward asthma and hay fever. The reply came: "Not if the osteopathic corrections are made properly along the spinal column, so that the whole of the lymph circulation is changed." (3109-1) According to his reading, excess toxins produced variations in lymph flow, becoming sluggish and less active in certain areas of his body, hence the need to have the entire lymph circulation altered.

After describing to one woman how the osteopath was to proceed step by step with specific adjustments, her reading concluded:

> These will aid in keeping tendencies for better distribution of that assimilated in the lymph and emunctory circulation, and also stimulate the cerebrospinal circulation of both blood supply *and* nerve energies; thus keeping the body attuned, keeping the activities for all the organs of the body nearer to their normal reactions.   1968-9

She was told to have these treatments about once a month, but it should be a *thorough* treatment, making for a gradual stimulation to specific areas.

Castor oil packs. One efficient and economical way of absorbing healing substances directly into body tissues is through packs. A rather unique use of castor oil in the form of packs is found in the Cayce readings: using wool flannel (a large enough piece to fold two to four thicknesses to be placed over the abdomen) saturated with cold-pressed castor oil, heating the oil first on a heating pad (with a plastic sheet or garbage bag between the pack and the pad). The pack, with the wool flannel against the skin, is then placed over the liver/gall duct area (right side of abdomen), the remainder of the pack covering the rest of the abdominal area. The wool flannel, plastic sheet, and heating pad (one on top of the other) can be held in place with a folded bath towel, tucked at your sides to stabilize the layers. A towel or plastic sheeting can also be placed underneath you to protect the bedsheets. Lie with the pack, as warm as tolerable, for one to one-and-a-half hours, resting, meditating, praying. Then remove the pack and cleanse the area with a washcloth, dipped in a cup of warm water into which a teaspoon of baking soda has been added. Store the pack in a glass jar or plastic container, leaving it in a cool place (kitchen cabinet, closet, or refrigerator). Castor oil is fairly stable, not turning rancid easily unless exposed for long periods of time to direct sunlight, so the pack can be reused a number of times. Add a fresh layer of the oil, about two tablespoons, to the pack at each reuse.

While a variety of sequences for the pack was given in the readings, the most common one and easy to follow was three days with the pack on, followed by four days off. Repeat the sequence for three weeks in a row, then skip a week. Following the fourth week (that is, on week five), you may want to repeat the on/off three-week cycle again, depending upon the condition you are experiencing.

One woman was given this advice (note the sequence and time differences suggested in her reading):

> ... begin with Castor Oil packs over the liver and the lacteal ducts area (over the pyloric end of the stomach itself and over this portion of the system). These we would keep two, three, four days, of two or three hours each day, until there is absorbed by the system from these hot packs sufficient for the activity of the lymph circulation to be increased through these areas.

Later in her reading, she asked:

> (Q) Did the radium treatment which I had over ten years ago leave any bad effects?
> (A) ... use the Castor Oil packs. Make for the increasing of the circulation in such measures and manners as to allow for the flow of the lymph circulation through the affected portions. . .   810-1

The next excerpt reminds us of the compatibility of two treatments—

namely, castor oil packs and abdominal massage—when used in conjunction with one another:

> On those days when the Castor Oil Packs are *not* given, we would—
> when ready to retire—massage across the whole of the abdomen with
> an equal combination of Olive Oil and Peanut Oil. Massage all the body
> will absorb, especially across the diaphragm area, over the liver and the
> caecum area, down the right side, you see, to the middle portion of the
> abdomen, or along the umbilical line or plexus. This will not only aid in
> making better absorption for the Castor Oil Packs but will add to the
> activity of the lymph circulation throughout the abdominal area.
>
> 1857-1

Usually, when the last castor oil pack (often the third one each week)
is taken, the readings suggested ingesting a small amount of olive oil
(from two teaspoons to half a teacup) to help empty the gall duct. Occasionally there were exceptions to this advice, as in the following, which
also noted the benefit of external/internal applications:

> The day following the packs, for the better eliminations through the
> alimentary canal, we would take internally the combination of properties
> found in Fletcher's Castoria. Taken in very small quantities will be much
> more effective; quarter to a half teaspoonful every half hour during the
> whole day. Do this each week on the day following the Castor Oil packs.
> This will create for the body the proper associations of the lymph
> circulation, that will be increased by the applications for those things
> without and from within; producing better peristaltic movement for the
> system, and bringing about bettered conditions for the body.   637-2

Increasing lymph circulation is one of the purposes of the castor oil
pack. Helping lymph to move may relieve problems later on; for example, poor lymphatic drainage of the heart may lead eventually to
tissue damage and even heart failure. When the lymph becomes slow
and sluggish, fluids begin to accumulate around cells, forcing them farther away from their source of nourishment, the blood capillaries. Because toxins are not being removed in a timely manner, some cells may

die, while others try to survive in their own waste products. Removal of waste is essential for better health. The Dead Sea, for example, is lifeless because it has no outlet; nothing grows around it and birds don't even fly over it, so it remains "dead." When the lymph flow is increased, however, the removal of poisons surrounding the cells is speeded up, swollen lymph nodes are reduced in size, and we generally feel more energized. This type of improvement, noted in the following excerpt, is also achieved with castor oil packs, again used in conjunction with other therapies:

> The effect of these oil packs is to enliven, through the activity of the absorption through the perspiratory system, the activities in such natures and measures as to produce a greater quantity (than at present) and a superficial activity of the lymph circulation; hence setting up drainages to such measures that the poisons will be eliminated from the system, through the application not only of other properties taken internally but in the use of the high enemas [colonics].   631-4

While much of the beneficial results of these packs remains largely anecdotal, the A.R.E. Clinic in Phoenix, Arizona, did two separate double-blind studies using the packs. A summary of the results, entitled "Castor Oil Packs: Scientific Tests Verify Therapeutic Value" by Harvey Grady, was reported in *Venture Inward* magazine. With only a minimal dose of a castor oil pack—a one-time-only two-hour treatment—results showed a significant increase in the total production of lymphocytes and T-11 cells than in the placebo group, representing a general boost in the body's defense status. Lymphocytes, you may recall from chapter 2, are the immune system's disease-fighting cells, which are produced and housed mainly in lymphatic tissue. Any improvement in our body's immune system would be a plus in our favor, and castor oil packs seem to provide this added benefit.

Heat. Generally, warm applications promote lymph flow as well as increase blood flow, but heat is contraindicated in cases of fever, acute infection, edema, recent injury, neuralgia, pregnancy, malignancy, ischemic conditions, pains of unknown origin, and so on.

There are various ways to apply heat to a body. *Diathermy*, a form of electrotherapy common in Cayce's day, produced heat in tissues and organs by using a high frequency electrical current, which could be regulated for the desired effect. Mentioned in chapter 5, diathermy was used by many doctors, principally osteopaths, and was also available in hospitals. There were three forms: long-wave, short-wave, and micro-wave, the first two being available in Cayce's time. Referring to the treatment as "deep therapy," the readings emphasized using a current of low frequency or low power. Its purpose was mentioned in the following: "the low electrical vibrations of the Diathermy [would] so heat the body as to cause the breaking up of the lymph disturbance . . . " (1761-1) In this case it was to be administered after [1761]'s third colonic, with the treatments about a week apart. It "heats the central portion of the nerve force in the low charge of electrical forces," another reading, 2541-5, states. Today diathermy is no longer available, according to the information in *An Edgar Cayce Home Medicine Guide*. Because of its interference with radio and TV stations, the therapy was discontinued.

To help "create a stimulation to that of the excretory system, especially through the sweat glands," a *vapor bath*—that is, a steam bath with a fume (vapor) added—was recommended for [3892]. Since these treatments were usually given at home with the person sitting above a steaming pot in a makeshift cabinet or covered up to the neck with a tentlike material, the fume itself—in this case a teaspoon of wintergreen—could be placed directly into the container: one-half pint of boiling water. "This will open the pores to such an extent that these will assist the lymphatic circulation in bringing the impurities through this portion of body in the manner that stimulates the system. Also keeping the alimentary canal in order . . . " (3892-1) Some health clubs and spas may offer such steam baths or cabinets.

A third heat application is the *salt rub* (mentioned under "Massage"), using coarse sea salt or Epsom salt, slightly mixed with water, and rubbing it over the skin. Mrs. [1300] asked for help in correcting the phlegm in her throat. She was advised to use an alkaline spray as well as receive massages. Then she was given this information about the effect of the salt rub:

The salt rub makes for an activity by the absorption through the skin, by the very influence of the heat and the cleansing of the pores of the body. Thus it absorbs those influences that create the inclinations for the lymph and superficial circulation to prevent proper coordination with the centers from which the cerebrospinal system receives its impulses.

Hence accumulations as phlegm, which arise from drainages from infectious forces in antrums and in the soft tissue of the nasal passages[,] will be *removed* from the body; not only by absorption and drainages, you see, and especially by or from the influence of cleansing the colon area, but by arousing the system to become less active in the acid forces and more free of the acid and the poisons. Thus we have the better condition.   1300-2

Sometimes referred to as a salt glow, a salt rub is basically a skin friction, recommended as a hydrotherapy treatment for people who have difficulty sweating or for general detox purposes. One man, after being given the suggestion for colonics followed by massages to help with eliminations, was told *not* to have salt rubs, "for the tendency will be to produce too *much* of an elimination, causing *more* irritation *to* that of the lymph circulation—or to the *capillary* circulation also." (5420-3) Caution and moderation are key principles in the Cayce health readings.

Radio-Active Appliance. This appliance, which has no connection whatsoever with radioactivity despite its name, is described as a type of battery that helps equalize the energy of the body by using the body's own current. A Circulating File, instruction booklets, and articles provide further explanations and descriptions of its use. Sold today as the Radiac®, this appliance is mentioned in more than eight hundred readings, being given as more of a preventative than a cure for serious illnesses.

One woman, suffering the effects of poor circulation and poor elimination, was told that the appliance equalizes "the circulation in the lymph and the nerve forces through the body." (3254-1) She was to meditate while using it. Another woman was advised to use the appliance while resting. "This will aid in causing a better balance . . . from the emunctories and the lymph circulation to the various lymph patches that cause this disturbance . . . " Her lymph centers were practically dissipated, the reading said, creating pressure in her adrenals and eventually giving her "a great deal of distress . . . " (3265-1) The relaxation effects of the appliance were also noted.

Asking about the weakness in her right eye, [987] was told that pressures in her upper dorsal and cervical spine created disturbances in her sensory system, affecting her hearing and taste as well. To create a balance, she was to use the appliance, circulating the attachments, as directed, around her body. "This keeps and produces the normal pull of the lymph *and* the impulse as created by the vibratory forces of the bodily functions." (987-3)

At times, various solutions can be used along with the appliance. One female chiropractor was told to use chloride of gold, as it "gives stamina to the center or plexus itself without taking it internally—that will raise for the circulatory system, especially the lymph, a *stamina* to the muscular forces so as to hold *all* muscular forces—yes, the *whole* body will be improved, you see." She asked questions about her prolapsed colon, a polyp on her uterus, and muscular contractions. In the latter case, she was told that the "muscular contraction is produced by the lack of coordination between the activity of the lymph with the urea in the circulation of the lymph and emunctories, see?" (701-1) (Urea, formed in the liver, is a waste product derived from the breakdown of protein; it is expelled from the body in the urine.) Then it went on to state a principal concept in the Cayce approach:

> This, then, makes for the natural correction, the normal correction . . . we are correcting the *cause* and nature corrects itself in the muscular contractions throughout the body. We remove the cause, we let nature make the corrections—for this is better than operative forces or any measures!   701-1

Nature works with the body's innate ability to heal itself. By focusing on the cause of an ailment and not necessarily the symptoms, we may assist and support this inner wisdom of the body. Of course, the physical body also builds up a resistance and allows other areas of the body to take up the slack or to carry out the hindered functions, as noted in this excerpt (found also in chapter 3):

One should consider that the *system* is builded to *resist* whatever may
arise, and it *takes that* direction in carrying out for what it *was*
constructed, and when it meets obstructions; then it attempts to build
around, or overcome, by *using* other portions or functionings to carry
out its function.   943-17

CONCLUSION

Of course, a number of other remedies were mentioned in individuals' readings—many of them only once—as being part of a regimen beneficial to their health and affecting the lymphatic system as well. Some
of them, as diathermy mentioned above, are unobtainable today (so
substitutes might have to be found), while others, such as tonics, tablets,
drugs, appliances, and compounds were specifically geared to the particular person alone. It is generally advisable, when choosing a remedy
or treatment that came from a specific reading, to consider going over
the entire text of the reading to acquaint yourself more fully with the
person's condition plus Cayce's description of the physiological processes taking place. If they are available, read the background notes (B),
which contain the inquiries made for a reading along with presenting
complaints and the questions to be answered in the reading, and the
reports (R), comprising the follow-up information, letters, doctors' sum-
maries, and further notes from Gladys Davis and others. Becoming well-
informed as to the nature of your illness and its process of development
will perhaps lead to a successful outcome, a healthy state of balance
and wellness.

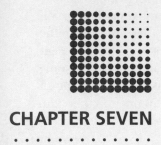

CHAPTER SEVEN
· · · · · · · · · · · · ·

The Wonders of Lymph

Like prospecting for gold, excavating and exploring the Cayce readings can lead to nuggets of insight, information, and intelligence. Hidden perhaps in unobtrusive sentences or paragraphs, these nuggets provide us with kernels of truth and wisdom that may surprise us and delight us. Several of these treasured pieces are presented here. While there is a variety of individual value in these excerpts, their importance may hinge on whether or not the physical condition alluded to is relevant to you personally. The excerpts presented below are not in any special order, yet it is hoped that they will offer further clarification and understanding—at least from the Cayce perspective—of the lymphatic system.

One particular danger in presenting any sort of overview of a specific bodily system is the tendency to overstress its importance. Of course, the lymph affects many physical processes and functions—elimination, circulation, immunity, digestion, and so forth—yet each of these systems, along with others, is important too. They all can be analyzed and researched, while explanations of each are thoroughly described in great detail in anatomy and physiology texts. The information from the readings is no doubt helpful and, to some extent, coincides with current scientific understanding; however, the descriptions of individuals' physical processes are some–times difficult to follow and comprehend. As we noted earlier, certain words may have a different meaning from the way they are used in the reading; also, it seems that at times Cayce himself is struggling to present the diagnosis as accurately and as clearly as possible. So here are some further insights from the Cayce readings that it is hoped may be of added benefit to you:

Physical Organisms and Spirit

The connections between spirit, mind and body are through the emunctory and the lymph flow in the body-force itself. It is at these places where there are physical hindrances that prevent a unified or coordinant activity when there is the attuning of the body [through meditation].   2946-4

. . . each cell in an organism is as a universe in itself, each attempting to manifest the purpose for which its functions are set in an organism, and should coordinate one with another . . .   433-1

. . . that which is good today . . . may be bad tomorrow. For what would be poison for someone, to another may be a cure. This is true in every physical organism.   1259-2

Lymph

Lymph is a circulation of blood . . . that forms by the mucous accumulations around or within lymph cells that were *protections* to the body, to prevent caking or hardening there.   687-1

. . . the lymph in its circulation . . . is controlled by the sympathetic system . . .   4163-1

. . . the area of the lymph and its closer circulation [is located] under arms, across portions of the body, the arm pits, the hands, in the groin, under knees, in the feet, and the like.   515-1

> . . . lymphatic centers [are] where lymphatic circulation comes closest
> to the surface.   282-1

> . . . lymphatic circulation comes close to the surface [in the] feet, under
> the knees, in the groin, in the sides, in and under the armpits, in the
> elbow, around the neck.   2351-1

Terms

Lymph is sometimes referred to as "water blood" (549-1) or "water of the blood" (389-3); sometimes the term "lymph blood" is also used (2455-2).

Leukocytes (also spelled "leucocytes"), white blood cells which are important to the body's defense system, are called "warriors of the system" (357-1), "warriors against inflammation" (1995-1), or "white blood" (568-2, 596-1, 808-15, 875-1, 974-1, 987-1, 1319-1, 1544-1, 3547-1, etc.), the latter being the designation for lymph itself in ancient times.

> . . . catarrh . . . means inflammation of the muco-membranes of the
> duodenum *and* intestines, see?   404-6

> . . . catarrhal condition is the lymph becoming so overcoated with the
> air in such measures or manners, not being properly balanced to
> produce the correct circulation.   681-2

> (Q) What do you mean by the fluids in the circulation?
> (A) The lymph circulation.   883-1

> . . . the centers in the blood supply . . . is where we change from the
> [venous] circulation to the vein circulation . . .   2483-1

> . . . phlegm . . . the *attempts* of the lymph to throw off or to meet the
> congestion [in the pulmonaries].   755-3

> . . . a lesion [is] an attempt of the blood flow (that is, the lymph and
> emunctory flow) to shield any injured portion or any pressure. This
> ofttimes increases the amount of pressure to other portions of the body.
>   1120-2

Adhesions are indicated, though these as we find—rather than true adhesions—are lymph that has become heavy, but not to the form that can be called lesions. Lesions would indicate that these had been adhered in such a manner as to become stationary.   1422-2

... lymph pockets [are] those protuberances that have produced the fire [from inflammation], as well as the sapping of the vitality and the strength of the body.   2047-1

... the lymph and emunctory circulation—that *is* the source through which *this* portion—that is, the alimentary canal, specific—receives its assimilated forces for its self-production.   2402-1

... calcium deposits [are a] crystallization of the conditions not eliminated, and these may be found in places or areas in the lymph circulation, as the nasal passages, at times in throat, in shoulder, the abdominal area close to the upper portion of the hips.   5273-1

... cohesions (that is, a closing of the intestinal tract itself in the caecum area), adhesions and lesions (that is, those tendencies for the intestines and the sac or covering of the intestines to adhere to the side or to the body itself) ...   533-2

... the emunctory circulation ... governs the eliminating properties within the body.   3879-1

... the liver ... is the secreting and excreting organ of the system, by which is purified most of the blood in the body.   4614-1

The white blood is the resistance in the body; the red blood is the rebuilding or the richness of the body, whereby we rebuild the wasted cells, or keep the body alive.   4614-1

... sleep is the building time of the physical forces to give and partake of rejuvenal expressions, both from circulation and from nerve tissue ...   5681-1

... foods in their digestion for the body are carried in the lacteal ducts
and the lacteals ...   433-1

... jejunum ... that portion of the intestinal system in which portions
of that digested or assimilated is carried back into the system.

5541-1

Stimulation of Lymph

(Q) How do I stimulate the lymph circulation?
(A) The lymph circulation—this is rather a broad question. The lymph
circulation is through various portions of the body itself, see? In
stimulating the lymph in the *alimentary canal,* of course it is usually
done by cathartics or such natures. [However, for this individual it would
be best done through diet.] But stimulate the gastric flows by the ganglia
along the cerebrospinal system that *govern the activity* of the organs as
related to the lymph flow in such a manner. In stimulating the lymph
flow for *ducts* through portions of the body, as in the glands about the
salivary activity from the mouth, stimulate the vagus centers and these
produce same as a flow through the system. These are differently
stimulated, you see, to produce lymph reaction. [Massage also stimulates lymph, the reading added.]   1140-2

... the increasing of the lymph flow [will] flush the congestion from the
system.   849-31

... keep the adhesions from forming—as much as practical—by the
stimulation of lymph flow through the areas where these tendencies
have been and are still indicated [upper lobe of liver to cecum area].

2153-10

Effects of Acidity

The harmful effects of an acidic condition are enumerated quite frequently in the readings. An acid diet causes "effluvium in the lymph
circulation that finds expression in an irritation to the superficial
circulation—or in the form of rash and pimples, and the irritations
over portions of the body." (566-9) How often do we associate skin

eruptions with what we've eaten?

> ... from the general tendency of acidity [has come] a slow activity; or the secretions from the liver and the lacteal activities produce a lack of the lymph circulation, so as to destroy a great deal of the peristaltic movement of the intestinal system. Hence we have a slowing of the activity, and at times disorders through the colon.   732-1

> Cold arises from overacidity and the tendency of the slowed circulation, or poor circulation, that has been indicated through the lymph circulation through the head and neck and face.   694-1

> A cold can't make headway when the warriors are sufficient, or the leucocytes!   386-3

> (Q) Why the occasional soreness in the region of my appendix?
> (A) There might be a soreness in almost any region with as much poison moving around in system!   481-1

> ... a tendency for acidity through the non-activity of the gall ducts ... makes the mucus membranes of the circulation to the head, through the secondary cardiac plexus area, susceptible to congestion or cold; which forms or produces an over supply of lymph to the bronchi and larynx area, producing an irritation that makes for a deep, hoarse or heavy cough [Here Mr. Cayce imitated the cough].   566-3

One woman, who became quite sleepy and suffered memory lapses whenever she tried to meditate or read, was told it was due to "toxic forces ... the poisons; and as the channels or centers through the lymph are opened, by concentration, the flow of lymph carries the tendency for drowsiness ... " (1152–10)

> ... the tendencies for an acidity through the very lymph flow itself [makes] the body susceptible to an increased circulation through the lymph flow of the head, the face and the throat.   1154-1

(Q) What causes gas around the heart?
(A) Excess acidity, produced by the overactivity of the amount of the influence for the *lymph* flow through these portions—or this is called upon and it produces gas.   1685-1

... there have been some indiscretions as to dampness of the feet; and with a little superacidity there is a severe contraction through the bronchi and the whole of the lymph for head, throat and bronchi.   1100-20

Not that there is not sufficient blood supply [anemia], but owing to the toxic forces there is the inclination for an impoverishment of the circulation as related to the *lymph*.   1224-3

An over alkalin condition is much worse even than a mild acidity; for an alkalin reaction easily dissolves certain tissue, while an acid condition usually attempts to create the effluvia about the lymph circulation as to reduce acidity.   437-6

Allergies

. . . the activities of the lymph and emunctory circulation, being charged—or through the allergies, cause the accumulations in any area where there are the larger patches of the emunctory or lymph bursa. There are a number of these patches, of course, in the feet, in hands, more than in other portions of the body, save in the soft tissue of lung and head and nasal passages.   3125-1

... those things and those elements, in the main, to which the body is allergic . . . must be kept low in the system; else these tendencies will also make for an irregular condition in the nerve forces as related to lymph and emunctory circulation.   257-243

Elimination Systems

Now remember, there are more than one channel of elimination! We eliminate through the drosses of the alimentary canal, we eliminate through the activities of the kidneys themselves, we eliminate through the very breath from the body. We eliminate from the activity of the lymph circulation, to the perspiratory system. And if these become clogged, any of these, either of the systems, then the other attempts to— of course—take care of the condition; but to the disturbing of some portion of the system.   601-22

. . . poisons, excesses of any nature, or drosses, are eliminated either through the alimentary canal, the activity of the kidneys and bladder, or are thrown off in the respiratory or perspiratory system. These arise from those variations produced in the flow of the lymph circulation . . .
                                                            3109-1

Those applications that have been made are very well, yet the condition continues—owing to not sufficient absorbing of the poisons and the inflamed portions, and the activity of the lymph flow to throw off and eliminate the poisons.   849-58

In the adjustments to be made, these are not so much corrections as to set up drainages, coordinating the areas . . . where there are the closer connection with the cerebrospinal and sympathetic nerve impulses; so that the drainages from the lymph as well as from the organic functions are carried off through the eliminating centers—alimentary canal, respiratory system, perspiratory system. These are the channels through which all of these used energies are to be eliminated.   3274-2

Through lack of proper eliminations there has been gradually builded such poisons or toxic conditions as to change the chemical reactions making for a lack of proper coordination between lymph circulation and the alimentary canal. Thus in segments and in muscular forces we find that poisons have crystallized, causing neuritic and arthritic pressures in the nerves and tendons of the body.   3559-1

. . . the food values should be digested and assimilated before entering into the large intestine or colon itself; for digestion or assimilation takes place throughout the system . . . and when there is the strain made on the lymph circulation through those portions of the colon that produces irritation there, it is like keeping scratching on a sore that doesn't heal properly. 440-18

Any of these [remedies] that make for increasing of the lymph circulation, will tend to make for a better elimination through the torso or through the lower portions of the body and their activity with the system.   515-2

When the eliminations through the alimentary canal are choked, either the liver or the kidneys, or both, suffer. So also does the lymphatic circulation, or the pulmonaries . . .   337-4

As is seen, in all bodies, not *all* eliminations are carried on *through* the alimentary canal . . . nearly fifty percent is eliminated through the activity of the hepatic circulation, but hepatic circulation—while *of* the liver and kidneys—may throw into the pulmonaries, or the lymphatic circulation, that which should have been carried off in other channels.   99-5

It is well that . . . the poisons as are not eliminated through the dross channel are thrown off. This, as seen, is the natural method—or nature's method—to prevent more destructive conditions in system . . .
                                                                                                                   4124-2

Immune Response

The swelling is the attempt of the body to meet the condition through producing sufficient of the hormones in the urea or the cellular forces from the leucocyte influence; to meet the accumulations of an impoverished circulation by a pressure. Thus swelling occurs, choking occurs, drippings occur at times when the reactions begin to set in—from the natural secretions that come from inflammation as may be created by such as an ordinary cold (as an illustration; not of the same nature), where tissue becomes involved and there are the attempts of the lymph to create an impulse to choke off the bacilli that attack the body in the soft tissues of throat or the nasal passages, or even the lung forces themselves.   1118-1

Tumors

. . . a double or quickening in the pulsation . . . is an ordinary indication that tumorous conditions exist in the system. Instead of there being the

skipping of a beat, it is at times as a *double* beat—even more than is
discernable in . . . pregnancy . . .   596-1

. . . tumors . . . are rather of the nature of lymph accumulations.

1319-1

. . . when there is any form of disturbance or infection in those areas
of the system [breast] where lymph glands form nobules, these may
gather in any of the glands of the body . . . If left alone, these may cause
such congestion in the mammary glands as to produce first a center
around which accumulations may gather, and thus cause those tendencies where a continual breaking down of resistances, and the inability
to eradicate same, might bring destructive forces.   1472-14

Swelling

. . . with the corrections in the lumbar and sacral area the circulation will
be more perfected and the coordination between the arterial and the
venous circulation will be better established, and overcome this
tendency for the lymph to produce the swelling in ankle and in limb.

604-1

. . . we have an accumulation in throat, in tonsil, in the adnoid area or
the back of the nasal cavity; the lymph tending to produce that of a
swelling nature, and these naturally become reservoirs for the accumulation of poisons that should be eliminated through the system.

671-1

(Q) What has produced the swelling to twice the normal size of leg?
(A) . . . the separation of the cells through the lymph and the superficial
circulation. And this involves the tissue throughout the limb.   988-6

. . . we find that a weak Mullein Tea would aid in reducing the tendencies
for the accumulation of lymph through the abdomen and the limbs.
Prepare same in this manner:
    To 1 pint of water add 1 ounce of the Mullein well bruised (with
some of the flower included, would be well). Let it come *almost* to a boil.

Then set it aside to cool. Keep it on ice, of course, and make fresh every day or two. Take a tablespoonful of this about twice or three times a day.
409-36

... the throwing of properties to be eliminated onto the kidneys has carried same (with this slowing of the hepatic circulation) into the lymph circulation. Thus the forming of not only splotches on the body but tendencies for swelling and inflammation in all areas where there is the circulation of the lacteal or lymph ducts ...   2289-5

... there are those tendencies in the present towards arthritic, neuritic-arthritic conditions, or lymph arthritis; which we find indicated in the swelling in joints of fingers, wrist, elbow, knees and feet at times.
935-3

... as to the amount of the uremic poisons that are allowed to reabsorb in the system, these cause an inclination for a dropsical effect ...
1888-1

(Q) What causes the swollen feet?
(A) Poor circulation in the lower portion of body, produced by pressure in the lower portion of sacral and lumbar region. Increased amount of lymphatic circulation.   4520-3

Coughs/Colds

The cough is the natural reaction from the poor circulation ... from there being a poor lymph circulation. The properties of the brandy with honey—but there should not be too *much* honey in same, but so the use of these may be active upon the gastric flow or the lymph circulation; and this will gradually be overcome.   632-7

(Q) How can I prevent chronic colds?
(A) Get rid of that which causes same! which is the general catarrhal condition that affects the superficial circulation, especially the lymph and the emunctory!   1601-1

[Colds] arise from over-acidity. When we keep a normal balance between the acids and alkalines for the body, we will find colds will be prevented. For, colds that are the more common to all bodies do not react in an alkaline condition. An alkalinity is destructive to colds. Hence any of those influences that may be had to alkalinize the body; not Alka-Seltzer but any of the citrocarbonates that make for the proper reactions to the lymph and the emunctory circulation will relieve cold. Citrus fruit juices taken occasionally, if there is the tendency for a cold, will create an alkalinity in the system such as to remove same.   1291-1

Owing to the presence of cold and congestion . . . the flow of lymph through the superficial circulation . . . causes a great deal of stiffness in the extremities, especially as indicated in the arms.   2526-2

(Q) What specific kind of shots should I take?
(A) Just take three cold shots. These are cold germs destroyed, then put in a tube and put into the body. It produces the effect of causing the lymph to create a greater quantity of leukocytes, which acts upon the system to increase circulation—thus keeping down cold. For it is the leukocyte that strangles each germ that enters, either through the nostril or the breath or by contamination. And the leukocyte must strangle same, so we increase it! If the circulation is slow, then there are not as many leukocytes. So we inject this type of serum to increase the quantity!   2528-4

Peristalsis

Applications were suggested throughout the readings "to create a better movement throughout the emunctory and lymph circulation, which is the activity that makes for the peristaltic movements through-out the intestinal system." (372-8)

(Q) Should the use of enemas be continued to aid in eliminations?
(A) Continue these until there is better peristaltic movement from the better flow of the lymph through intestinal system.   641-7

. . . an over acidity of the lymph in the digestive system [takes] away from the elasticity of the peristaltic movement of the intestinal tract itself.

2176-1

Laxatives

Laxatives were considered severe to the body (1561–22). They were also known to strain the lymph circulation (654–5).

. . . as a laxative we would find Eno Salts preferable to so much of those that act as only a stimul[us] to the emunctory and lymph circulation through the intestinal system and thus producing a strain on an already overtaxed condition in the liver.

667-7

The Senna tea is better than the Syrup of Senna . . . the regular senna tea—made from the senna pods or leaves—will get better drainage and better activity in the association with the drying effect upon the lymph . . . made rather strong . . . at least a good teacup full.

1553-27

Enemas are not straining if taken properly. They are preferable, much preferable, much more easy upon the body than so much laxatives that only take from the system the vitality that should be strengthening in lymph circulation. For an eliminant, *any* eliminant, is an exciting of the mucous membranes to activity.

1242-2

. . . enemas are preferable to the eliminants that cause a reaction through the system or an exercising of the lymph and mucous membrane activities. These are well to be taken but do not depend upon these; just take them occasionally. Depend rather upon the activities of the assimilating system, and as these are built up we would find all of the disturbances gradually disappearing.

1259-2

Drying Conditions

That a drying condition will eventually become inflamed (264–55; 549–1) is mentioned in several readings. Senna tea was considered good for this so-called drying effect (1553–27).

. . . the lack of circulation, by so much blood supply being taken up in

the lymph and the serums of system . . . makes for a dryness . . . Dry
catarrhal condition.   5439-1

No sign of cancer . . . though there is a lack of sufficient lymph circulation.
Hence . . . there is the tendency for dryness. Thus the use of the
massage . . .   2390-4

(Q) What can I do to overcome constipation?
(A) . . . first by the eliminating of some of the sources that tend to dry
or call on the lymph to be used in other portions and not through the
alimentary canal. Do have at least the three or four colonics indicated.
Then with the diet and with the massages, this should be well improved.
                                          2801-6

. . . through the colon itself there is caused inflammation that tends to
produce in the fecal forces a drying, or lack of the proper activity, of the
lymph flow through this portion of the digestion.   1223-1

. . . there is a form of congestion which is of the nature as to cause the
drying of tissue in those areas where there are the needs for the greater
excesses of lymph and emunctory circulation . . .   2059-1

. . . the drying of the lymph flow through the colon . . . caused a clogging.
                                          2308-2

(Q) Is there any physical abnormality of the intestines?
(A) Only the effect of sedatives and the lack of natural flow of the lymph
that is dried by same and the tendencies for adhesions through
alimentary canal. [Gentle massages and castor oil packs were recommended.]   3398-2

Accumulation of Lymph

. . . too great a quantity of lymph . . . gathers in those portions of the
system. Equalizing the circulation, changing the activities through the
diet, the digestive system . . . will relieve these distresses [pain in back].
                                          734-1

If temperature arises in the body, reduce same by the colonic irrigations—that we may remove the tendency for this plethora in the lymph accumulations.   787-1

The gallstones are not the main disorder. While they appear in that area indicated, this is from accumulations of lymph pockets.   2956-2

... a lymph accumulation in the various portions of the system ... makes for dullness in activity, or lack of the return of vital forces after periods of rest ...   685-1

The natural tendency for the overflow of the lymph to adjust the body causes plethora conditions in the abdominal cavity, but these disappear as the blood or the circulation adjusts itself.   1034-1

... too much of the lymph appears in portions of the system. This [is] a hindrance in the circulation ...   1278-1

... by an excess of lymph and emunctory circulation ... many portions of the body as related to organic functioning have become so engorged as to produce a great excess of poisons in the system.   1355-1

... the attempt of the hepatic circulation to adjust itself without the proper functioning of the liver has made for a greater accumulation of the lymph ...   1850-1

... inflammation [causes] those accumulations of lymph through the superficial and internal parts of the body.   3093-1

There are times when the circulation becomes too much; carrying to the outer portions of the skin too much lymph and cause too much secretions. Then we have the effect of pus ...   5605-1

Activity of Lymph

... from the very source of infection, through the very lymph flow, conditions are produced in other portions of the body ...   1485-1

. . . the organs of assimilation; the pancreas, the liver, the gall duct . . .
are governed primarily or principally through the lymph and the
sympathetic circulation.   1506-2

. . . the flow—or activity of digestion—is carried on through the nerve
forces' activity upon the lymph circulation. Thus there is the tendency
to swell, or to form gas—because of the excess acids in the wrong portion
of the system.   1506-2

. . . when there is the inclination for the lack of proper eliminations,
accumulations of poisons hinder the lymph from carrying into the
rebuilding forces of the body the new or full blood supply . . .
                                                                      1620-3

[This condition] is rather the inflammation of the covering of the bone
itself in the areas where joints themselves are, as it were, "oiled" by
lymph.   3547-1

(Q) Why the temperature?
(A) . . . the attempt of the lymph circulation to create sufficient of
destructive forces that will make for the accumulations to carry on
through the healing forces of the body.   759-12

. . . the lymph and the tissue weakest in system receives or takes on the
conditions produced by the toxins left by the poor eliminations.
                                                                      779-8

. . . lymph that has become, as it were, inflamed . . . becomes
interpenetrating to portions of the system where slowed circulation has
or does become indicated by the general activities of the body.
                                                                      849-13

. . . *any* condition that overtaxes the nerve plexuses [will] cause a drain
on the lymph circulation, and through same obtains, as it were, the
poisons in the system by re-absorption.   900-273

(Q) What causes gurgling around the area of the water tumor in pelvis? (A) This is the system gradually absorbing or making for the lymph flow through same.   1152-5

. . . the tendency for inflammation that arises and temperature that comes at times [produces] an increase of flow of the lymph circulation to cause a greater reaction.   1190-1

. . . all portions of the superficial activity of the lymph circulation [are] affected by the activity of this particular functioning of the [thyroid] gland [growth of nails, hair, and cuticle].   1490-1

The tendencies for poisons through various portions of the system indicate that some of these have been picked up or distributed through the body, through the lymph circulation . . .   1992-5

This seepage or inflammation in structural portions causes in the extremities, through the lymph circulation, a tingling or trembling akin to what might be called tic . . .   2204-1

. . . the lymph and the blood supply are able to destroy and rebuild cellular tissue in blood stream. This gives new life, or renew life to tissue in the nerve system, especially sympathetic, and adds to the resistance of the physical forces in body.   2233-2

[The] slowing of the lymph through the circulation in the abdominal area causes an engorgement in the ascending and a part of the transverse colon . . .   2388-1

There are those tendencies for the thinning of the walls of the lymph flow through the body, owing to the tendency of the body to carry impurities that should have been eliminated through their normal channels . . .   2392-3

. . . the blood receives impulses—through activities of organs supplied by glandular influence in those organs, or in glands themselves—

through which portions of the lymph and emunctory activity produce a plasm that is to become active in the muscular forces, the nerve tissue, the tendons and the replenishing or rebuilding of the organs them-selves.   2546-1

. . . digestion takes place through that absorbed and carried by the lymph and the hepatic circulation . . . to the body as food values.
                                        5632-1

. . . there have been leakages in the intestinal tract from thinned walls . . . so that the absorption—or the lymph and emunctory circulation, carry much of that as should be eliminated through other channels.
                                        5557-1

. . . the system in attempting to prevent spreading [of poisons] created segregation by the accumulations of the lymph and the leucocyte about same.   487-23

As the lymph from the white blood is thrown around the bacilli they are drawn off and expelled.   538-1

Lymph Antiseptic

The occasional use—when this [phlegm] occurs—of a gargle with Lavoris or Glyco-Thymoline will materially aid. This does not injure; and is a good intestinal as well as lymph antiseptic, and will be beneficial. It is alkaline reacting also. So if small quantities are swallowed, it is beneficial, not harmful.   808-15

Scar Tissue

. . . injections that were given as a preventative [have] caused tissue to become involved and to form in the lymph and the capillary circulation what is termed scar tissue.   1363-1

With the formation of cold [several years ago], there was an accumula-tion in the lymph circulation that formed an adhesion; and this eventually produced a layer of scar tissue.   2758-1

Massage

... the Swedish massage ... is for the superficial circulation, to keep attunement as it were between the superficial circulation or the lymph and the exterior portion with the activities of the body. These treatments should not be hurried, and there should be given sufficient period for the reaction to the body.   1158-11

(Q) What causes and what may be done for the swelling of face, especially under eyes?
(A) The massage in the shoulders and the neck should allay, or bring about better lymph circulation.   2491-4

At least every other day there should be ... not the heavy therapy but a gentle massage that would stimulate the activity of the ganglia at each center along the spinal system, as well as stimulating of the ganglia in the frontal portions of the body—of the lymph centers—as to distribute this energy through the system.   3099-1

Hydrotherapy

[Hot baths] take *from* the system those excesses of poisons and accumulations in the capillary and lymph circulation... *especially* those carrying the Epsom Salts ... taken as sitz baths occasionally. 2225-1

[Steam baths with Atomidine] produce to the superficial circulation sufficient of the opening of the pores that there may be an absorption to the superficial circulation and the lymph as it works through same the properties to produce a healing *and* a coordination in that portion of the system.   1762-1

Food for Lymph

... include [in the diet] the very strengthening blood and lymph building foods—as beef juices (not soups, but juices) and liver juices. 2639-1

In the matter of the diet—do have oft ... those properties that carry a great deal of iodine and calcium; or sea foods often. Those that carry the elements indicated especially in beets and beet tops. These are healing

in their activity upon the lymph circulation. They are even capable of
destroying certain characters of bacilli in the system.   3056-1

. . . any of carbonated waters or strong drinks of any kind, especially
anything with hops . . . tend to produce a filling of the lymph through the
alimentary canal, as well as the lymph flow in throat. Don't use these
things.   3534-1

. . . Atomidine . . . will add iodine to the system that is assimilated with
the system . . . and adds to the ability of the lymph and the muco-
membranes of the system to secrete proper secretions for the functioning of organs . . .   3988-1

Noons—rather the full green vegetable salad, with or *without* the
dressings—alternate at times to suit the taste, or there may be made a
dressing of lemon juice with paprika, or such, that makes for a stimul[us]
to the glands or ducts of the *digestive* glands of the system, particularly
those of the lacteals, that the gastric juices with the stimuli to the system
may not be *over* burdening, but keeping an even balance in same. Keep
the mental attitudes properly in their seasons, especially when supplying food for the resuscitating of the system, and *seeing*—as it is taken—
that as *is* to be accomplished *by* that taken, *knowing* what each property
is to supply to the system, and see it being accomplished.   255-10

CONCLUSION

Having even a little knowledge and understanding about the functioning of our physical bodies gives us insight into how we can help
keep ourselves in optimal health. The role that the lymph plays is a
major part in this process, a theme running throughout the Cayce health
information. Knowledge is power, an old proverb states. So with this
basic introduction to the lymphatic system, we have the power to make
those changes and follow those paths that will lead us to a healthful
balance and harmony that is our purpose in life.

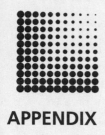

APPENDIX

The content of this book covers primarily information from the Edgar Cayce readings on lymph, yet it would be beneficial to the reader to be acquainted with some non-Cayce applications as well. While a number of these resources exist, one will be presented here: the Dr. Vodder method of Manual Lymph Drainage (MLD®).

Named after a husband–and–wife team, the Vodder method of Manual Lymph Drainage had its beginnings in the 1930s in the south of France, where Emil and Estrid Vodder, massage therapists, were working at a physical therapy institute in Cannes. Many of their clients were British citizens recovering from chronic colds with accompanying swollen lymph neck nodes. One day a client came in for treatment suffering from a nose and throat infection, migraine headaches, and blemished skin. Emil theorized that a blockage in the lymph nodes was the cause of the infection. After palpating the hard, swollen cervical nodes, he "saw" with eyes closed the lymph node chains that act as a drainage for all the organs and nodes in the head and neck. Convinced early on in his professional career that the body should be regarded as a whole, he began to work intuitively and use his knowledge of anatomy to formulate a new set of massage techniques specifically for compromised lymph systems. Using gentle, rotary motions lightly over the skin, he was able to cure his patient successfully. Palpating the skin with further circular pumping and draining actions accompanied by light pressure, the skin was moved and stretched exactly along the lymph pathways—unless there was a blockage; in which case, the fluid could be shunted around it. He began to treat many different ailments using this therapy, realizing that obstructed, malfunctioning lymph nodes could lead to a host of ailments and symptoms.

Continuing their research and study, the Vodders eventually presented their findings at a "Health and Beauty" exhibition in Paris in 1936. It was a success. But the outbreak of World War II later intervened, and they were forced to return to their native Denmark and start over, founding a new MLD institute in Copenhagen. Continuing to give lectures and courses, they slowly made inroads into other countries, and interest in their work gradually increased, bolstered by research and new technology. They regarded the lymph system as the source of life. Not only does it serve to clean tissues through drainage, but it also protects and defends the physical body, carrying out vital functions.

Research continues to demonstrate the method's effectiveness, pointing out that classical massage techniques had no drainage effects whatsoever. Pressure and movement were shown to be key elements in producing results—hence the importance of learning the exact and proper technique through correct training. It is not specifically a massage technique but a completely new manual method for working with the superficial lymph, which lies just below the skin surface, and using light pressure, along with subtle hand movements, to move this fluid.

Training consists of four levels: a basic course and three therapy courses. Basic and Therapy I are forty hours each; Therapy II and III are taught together in a two-week-long session, adding Combined Decongestive Therapy to the curriculum. With the passing of several exams, students become MLD therapists and are required every two years to do a twenty-five-hour MLD Review, in which they update and fine-tune their skills plus keep current with ongoing research. The technique is widely accepted in Europe. The Vodder Clinic in Walchsee, Austria, established in 1972, continues to carry on the Vodders' work, while the Dr. Vodder School™—International, located in Victoria, British Columbia, Canada, which opened in the late 1970s, also provides training in this method.

In the foreword to the Wittlingers' *Textbook*, Dr. Vodder mentions a prophecy made in the 1940s by one of the first lymph researchers in the

U.S., Professor Cecil Drinker, stating that the lymph system would eventually be recognized as the most important organic system in humans and in animals. With the rapid scientific progress made in this field and the increased awareness of its importance, it seems that that prophecy is close to being fulfilled.

Glossary

Abrasion—a scraping, wearing away, or rubbing off (e.g., skin); a spot rubbed bare of skin or mucous membrane

Adhesion—fibrous tissue that abnormally joins body parts or tissues that are normally separate; usually the result of inflammation

Adiron—also called Codiron; contains cod liver oil; source of vitamins A, B, D, E, and G

Agar—gelatinous product extracted from seaweed; laxative and gelling agent used in cooking

Alimentary canal—gastrointestinal (GI) tract; a continuous, hollow, muscular tube that winds through the body from mouth to anus

Anemia—condition in which there is a reduction in the number or volume of red blood corpuscles

Antrum—sinus cavity in upper jaw; a cavity

Appendix—fingerlike projection from the large intestine; also called vermiform appendix

Arterioles—small arteries

Artery—blood vessel carrying blood away from the heart

Arthritis—inflammation of a joint or joints

Ascites—fluid that accumulates in the tissue spaces and organs in the abdominal cavity

Assimilation—capacity to utilize food; body's performance of the complicated metabolic processes of digestion and elimination

Asthenia—weakness; loss of strength or energy

Asthma—condition of the lungs characterized by decrease in diameter of some air passages; sufferer has mild or severe attacks of difficulty in breathing

Atomidine—iodine from one percent of iodine trichloride; "atomic iodine"; taken orally in small quantities; each drop supplies about six times the minimum daily requirement of iodine; an easily assimilated form of iodine

Autoimmune—resulting from the immune system reacting against the body's own tissues

Avascular—not vascular; containing no vessels

Bladder—bag in the pelvic cavity that holds urine flowing from the kidneys

Boils—tender, swollen areas caused by staphylococcal infection around hair follicles

Bone marrow—spongy, porous material found in center of bone; produces red blood cells

Bright's disease—disease of the kidneys; chronic form of glomerulo-nephritis

Bursa (pl., bursae)—fluid-filled sac that provides cushioning between adjacent areas that otherwise might rub against each other

Capillary—smallest blood vessel; serves as crossing point between arterioles (small arteries) and venules (small veins)

Cartilage—tough white flexible tissue attached to bones; gristle; has no blood vessels

Castor oil—colorless or yellowish oil obtained from the bean or seed of the castor-oil plant

Catarrh—inflammation of mucous membranes, usually in nose and throat areas, causing an increase in flow of mucus

Cathartics—medicines that stimulate bowel evacuation; purgatives

Cecum (also spelled caecum)—pouch that is the beginning of the large intestine, located at the junction of the small and large intestines

Cervical—referring to the neck (as in vertebrae)

Chiropractic—science and art of restoring or maintaining health by employing manipulation of the body joints, especially of the spine, to restore normal nerve function

Chyle—milk-white fluid formed in the small intestine; "juice"; composed of lymph and emulsified fats

Chyme—digested food in the small intestine

Cimex lectularius—homeopathy remedy recommended for dropsy; made from bedbug juice

Citrocarbonate—a proprietary antacid and alkalizer

Coagulation—blood clotting; a clumping, thickening, or congealing

Coco-quinine—cocoa butter and quinine; remedy for various topical infections; mosquito and insect repellant

Cod liver oil—oil made from the liver of cod fish and other related fishes; rich in vitamins A and D

Cohesion—a closing of the intestinal tract itself in the caecum area (Cayce readings); tendency to stick together

Colonic—high enema; also called colonic irrigation

Constipation—difficult or infrequent evacuation of fecal material from the large intestine

Coordination—harmonious action; skillful and balanced movement of different parts; in the Cayce readings it is often referred to as the balance between the cerebrospinal and peripheral nervous systems

Crews lymph pump—respiratory pump (mentioned in the Cayce readings)

Cuticle—outer layer of skin; epidermis; hardened skin, such as base and sides of fingernail

Cyst—abnormal sac or capsule containing a semisolid material, a liquid, or a gas; closed epithelium-lined sac with a distinct membrane; four types: retention, exudation, embryonic, and parasitic; usually harmless but may become malignant

Cystitis—inflammation of the bladder

Diaphragm—dome-shaped muscle forming the bottom of the thoracic cage

Diathermy—treatment to provide heat, using a current of low frequency; both short- and long-wave methods available in Cayce's time

Dobell's solution—wash or spray to treat nasal and throat diseases; liquid consisting of sodium bicarbonate, borax, phenol, and glycerin

Domino effect—theory that a certain result will follow a certain cause

Dross—waste matter; worthless stuff; impurities; rubbish

Eczema—dermatitis; inflammation of upper layer of skin; characterized by blotches, redness, itching, scaling, and swelling

Edema—an abnormally large amount of fluid that accumulates in connective tissue, intercellular spaces of the body, or in body cavities; also called dropsy

Effluvium—a smell, odor, or fume that is unpleasant; originates from waste or decaying matter

Eliminant—substance that helps to expel waste from the body; an evacuating remedy

Emunctory—any organ or body part that gives off waste products, such as the kidneys, lungs, or skin; (adj.) excretory

Endothelial—made up of simple squamous cells which line the inner surfaces of the circulatory organs and other closed cavities

Enema—insertion of liquid into the rectum through the anus by means of a syringe, usually for treatment of constipation

Engorged—congested; distended or swollen with fluids

Eno salts—laxative powder

Erysipelas—acute infectious disease of skin or mucous membranes, caused by streptococcus; characterized by oval patches which enlarge and spread, becoming red, swollen, and tender; a form of cellulitis

Eustachian tube—a slender tube between the middle ear and the pharynx; helps to equalize air pressure in the eardrum

Exhalation—breathing out

Femur—thighbone

Fever—elevation of body temperature

Fletcher's Castoria—laxative often used for children; made from a natural vegetable ingredient

Gallstones—small, hard particles that form in the gallbladder owing to infection or blockages

Ganglia—masses of nerve cells running parallel to the spine (sing., ganglion)

Gastric—pertaining to the stomach

Glyco-Thymoline—an alkalizing formula primarily used as a spray or gargle for nasal and throat passages; also used as an eye wash, in packs, as an intestinal antiseptic, and for sunburn; available at the time of Cayce as well as today

Growth—anything that grows; any abnormal mass or proliferation of tissue (e.g., tumor); abnormal formation

Hay fever—common allergy characterized by itching, watery eyes and sneezing; largely a reaction to pollen and mold spores

Hepatic—referring to the liver; in the Cayce readings, kidneys, bladder, heart, and lungs are included; it is divided into upper and lower hepatic (several of these organs are included in one or the other)

Hodgkin's disease—characterized by progressive enlargement and inflammation of lymphoid tissues, especially the spleen

Homeostasis—tendency to uniformity or stability in normal body states; maintenance of relatively stable conditions in a system by internal processes that counteract any departure from the normal

Humor—body fluid; any of four fluids (blood, phlegm, choler, melancholy) formerly considered responsible for one's health and disposition

Hydrotherapy—treatment of disease by use of water

Ileocecal valve—section where the ileum of the small intestine joins the large intestine

Infection—invasion of the body by harmful microorganisms

Infectious—liable to be transmitted by infection or inflammation

Inhalation—breathing in

Intercostal—muscles between the ribs; helps lungs to inflate

Interstitial—fluid found in between the cells

Jejunum—middle section of the small intestine (situated between the duodenum and ileum); absorbs nutrients from digested food

Kidneys—pair of organs that removes waste products from the blood; secretes urine

Knot—any knoblike swelling; usually firm to the touch; hard lump, swelling, or protuberance in or on a part of the body or a bone or a process

Lacteals—specialized lymphatic capillaries of the small intestine; absorbs fats and other nutrients

Large intestine—final section of digestive tract, consisting of ascending, transverse, descending, and sigmoid colon; bowel

Lesion—harmful change in the tissue of a body organ, caused by injury or disease

Leukocyte—(also spelled "leucocyte") white blood cells important to the body's defense system

Lipids—fats

Liver—large organ in abdomen; secretes bile; concerned with metabolism, blood clotting, and protein manufacture

Lumbago—pain in lumbar region of the back

Lump—any abnormal swelling; a piece or mass of indefinite shape and size

Lungs—main organs of respiration lying within the chest cavity behind the rib cage

Lymph—a clear, yellowish, or colorless fluid, resembling blood plasma; found in the intercellular spaces and in the lymphatic vessels of vertebrates; formed in the tissue spaces throughout the body; carried by lymphatic vessels to central area of body where it is combined with the blood supply; white (watery) portion of blood; part of nerve circulation (Cayce readings)

Lymphangion—section of the lymphatic vessel between two valves; "lymph heart"

Lymphatic system—cleanses the body's internal structure; involved with immunity and fat absorption; composed of lymph, lymphatic vessels, lymph nodes, Peyer's patches, and lymphatic organs

Lymphatic vessel—structures which carry lymph; lymphatics

Lymphitis—technically, inflammation of the lymph (Cayce readings)

Lymph nodes—oval or bean-shaped structures scattered throughout the body in group clusters; purification and filtering centers for lymph

Lymphocyte—type of white blood cell produced in lymphatic tissue; disease-fighting cells

Manual lymph drainage therapy—passive compression of the body's soft tissues

Massage—a rubbing and kneading of the body to stimulate circulation and relieve tension; usually done with the hands

Mercury Quartz Light—sunlamp

Milk of Bismuth—an absorbent; prevents toxins from irritating the mucous membranes (Cayce readings)

Milk of Magnesia—a milky-white fluid used as a laxative and an antacid

Mucus—(adj., mucous) lubricating material excreted from membranes in gastrointestinal tract and sinus cavities

Mullein stupes—poultices made from fresh mullein leaves; applied with gauze or cloth to swollen areas, such as varicose veins; herb can also be used as a tea to improve lymph circulation (Cayce readings)

Neuralgia—severe pain along the course of a nerve; a form of neuritis

Neurasthenia—nervous prostration

Neuritis—nerve inflammation; inflammation of a nerve that attacks peripheral nerves

Osteopathy—treatment of disease and abnormalities by manipulating bones and muscles

Peripheral nerves—nerves that link the brain and spinal cord with muscles, skin, organs, and other parts of the body

Peristalsis—wavelike, rhythmic movement of food through the alimentary canal by muscular contractions

Peyer's patches (glands)—collections of lymphatic tissue located in the submucosa of the ileum (small intestine); they help to confine infectious material and prevent bacteria from penetrating the intestinal wall

Phlegmatic temperament—"lymphatic"; not easily excited; sluggish; apathetic

Pimples—small, inflamed spots on the skin

Plasma—colorless fluid part of blood in which corpuscles are suspended

Plethora—the state of being too full; overabundance; excess; an abnormal condition characterized by an excess of blood in the circulatory system or in some part of it

Pleurisy—inflammation of the pleura (membrane that covers the lungs) owing to either bacterial or viral infection

Plexus—network of nerves or blood vessels or lymphatic glands

Pocket—any small bag or pouch; cavity, sac, or enclosure that holds something

Psoriasis—skin disease characterized by red, scaly patches

Pyloric—distal end of stomach

Radio-Active Appliance—type of battery, but with no measurable electric charge; seems to affect the body's electrical energies (Cayce readings)

Radium Water—treatment for cancer and various disorders

Right lymphatic duct—one of the main lymphatic vessels through which lymph passes into the venous blood

Roseola—rose-colored rash

Saffron tea—herb used primarily for its perspiration-inducing quality and as a digestive aid; also known as Yellow or American Saffron

Sal soda—washing soda

Salt rub—sea salt or Epsom salts, slightly mixed with water, then rubbed over the body as a skin friction; also called salt glow

Sciatic lumbago—low back pain

Senna tea—herb whose leaves are used in teas as a laxative

Serous fluid—thin, yellowish fluid that remains from blood when the rest has clotted

Sinusitis—inflammation of the lining of the sinus cavities

Small intestine—body's main digestive organ where food is chemically broken down for use in body's cells

Spleen—organ at the left of the stomach; involved in maintaining proper condition of the blood; manufactures, stores, and destroys blood cells

Subcutaneous—under the skin

Submucosa—a layer of connective tissue located beneath a mucous membrane

Swelling—any abnormal enlargement of a body part

Sympathetic—superficial circulation, of lymph and emunctory nature (Cayce readings); part of the autonomic nervous system which stimulates the body to prepare for action

Systemic—affecting the whole

Taut—tense

Thoracic—dorsal; between head or neck and abdomen; chest

Thoracic duct—one of the main lymphatic vessels where lymph passes into the venous blood

Thymus—glandular structure in chest near base of the neck

T lymphocyte—white blood cell; helps protect against viral infections; detects and destroys some cancer cells

Tonsil—mass of special lymph tissue; one of two small organs at sides of throat near root of the tongue

Tonsillitis—infection or inflammation of the tonsils

Toris compound—laxative preparation

Toxemia—condition in which bacterial products or poisonous substances (toxins) are spread throughout the body via the bloodstream

Tumor—swelling; new growth of tissue in which cell multiplication is uncontrolled and progressive; new and actively growing tissue; abnormal benign or malignant mass of tissue, arising without obvious cause from cells of preexistent tissue; growth of faster than normal tissue; classified according to origin and whether it is malignant or benign; has no physiologic use or function

Ureter—tube that drains urine from the kidneys into the bladder

Urethra—duct by which urine is discharged from the bladder to the outside

Uric acid—waste product present in blood and excreted in the urine

Uricacidemia—accumulation of uric acid in the blood

Urine—waste liquid that collects in the bladder and is discharged from the body; fluid end product of kidney activity

Usoline—also known as Nujol or mineral oil or Russian White Oil

Vein—blood vessel carrying blood to the heart

Ventriculin—powder taken orally to stimulate formation of reticulocytes (type of red blood cell)

Venules—small veins

Vertebra—single bone or segment of the spinal column (pl., vertebrae)

Villi—minute, hairlike, fingerlike projections that cover the mucous membrane lining of the small intestine

Violet Ray machine—a high voltage, low amperage source of static electricity; hand-held device with various types of glass applicators

Viscera—organs within body

Wet-Cell Appliance—a battery producing a very small but measurable electric current; stimulates growth of nerve tissue (Cayce readings)

Zilatone—laxative compound

Bibliography

American Medical Association Home Medical Encyclopedia, The. (Two volumes). New York, N.Y.: Random House, Inc., 1989.

Bantam Medical Dictionary, The. Rev. ed. New York, N.Y.: Bantam Books, 1981.

Bisacre, Michael, Richard Carlisle, et al, eds. *The Illustrated Encyclopedia of the Human Body.* New York, N.Y.: Exeter Books, 1984.

Bolton, Brett, compiler. *Foods for Health and Healing.* Virginia Beach, Va.: A.R.E. Press, 1997.

Buchman, Dian Dincin. *The Complete Book of Water Therapy.* New Canaan, Conn.: Keats Publishing Inc., 1994.

Carter, Mary Ellen, and William A. McGarey, M.D. *Edgar Cayce on Healing.* New York, N.Y.: Warner Books, Inc., 1972.

Chaitow, Leon. *Hydrotherapy: Water Therapy for Health and Beauty.* Boston, Mass.: Element Books, Inc., 1999.

Chikly, Bruno, M.D. *Dissection of the Human Lymphatic System.* (VCR; two tapes). Palm Beach Gardens, Fla.: International Alliance of Healthcare Education, 1999.

————. *Lymph Drainage Therapy I Study Guide. Lymphatic Pathways: Anatomical Integrity.* Palm Beach Gardens, Fla.: The Upledger Institute, Inc., 1996.

————. *Silent Waves: Theory and Practice of Lymph Drainage Therapy.* Scottsdale, Ariz.: I.H.M. Publishing, 2001.

Clark, John O.E., ed. *A Visual Guide to the Human Body.* New York, N.Y.: Barnes and Noble, 1989.

Crouch, James E., Ph.D. *Functional Human Anatomy.* 3rd ed. Philadelphia, Penn.: Lea & Febiger, 1978.

Dorland, W.A. Newman, A.M., M.D., F.A.C.S. *The American Illustrated Medical Dictionary.* 22nd ed. Philadelphia, Penn.: W.B. Saunders Company, 1951.

Duggan, Joseph and Sandra. *Edgar Cayce's Massage, Hydrotherapy, and Healing Oils.* Virginia Beach, Va.: Inner Vision Publishing Company, 1989.

Duggan, Sandra, R.N. *Edgar Cayce's Guide to Colon Care.* Weymouth, Mass.: Inner Vision Publishing Company, 1995.

Edgar Cayce Home Medicine Guide, An. Virginia Beach, Va.: A.R.E. Press, 1982.

Földi, M., M.D., and R. Strössenreuther, M.D. *Foundations of Manual Lymph Drainage.* 3rd ed. St. Louis, Mo.: Elsevier Mosby, 2005.

Földi, Michael, M.D., and Ethel Földi, M.D. *Lymphoedema: Methods of Treatment and Control.* (English translation). Upper Beaconsfield, Victoria, Australia:

Lymphoedema Association of Victoria, 1993.

Furst, Jeffrey. *The Over-29 Health Book.* Norfolk, Va.: Donning, 1979.

Gabbay, Simone, R.N.C.P. *Nourishing the Body Temple: Edgar Cayce's Approach to Nutrition.* Virginia Beach, Va.: A.R.E. Press, 1999.

————. *Visionary Medicine: Real Hope for Total Healing.* Virginia Beach, Va.: A.R.E. Press, 2003.

Grady, Harvey. "Castor Oil Packs: Scientific Tests Verify Therapeutic Value." *Venture Inward* (July/August 1988), pp. 12–15.

Gray, Henry, F.R.S. *Gray's Anatomy.* Rev. Am. ed. New York, N.Y.: Bounty Books, 1977.

Guinness, Alma E., ed. *ABCs of the Human Body: A Family Answer Book.* Pleasantville, N.Y.: The Reader's Digest Association, Inc., 1987.

Guyton, Arthur C., M.D. *Anatomy and Physiology.* New York, N.Y.: Saunders College Publishing, 1985.

Harris, Robert. "An Introduction to Manual Lymph Drainage: The Vodder Method." *Massage Therapy Journal.* Evanston, Ill.: American Massage Therapy Association, Winter 1992.

Hildreth, Arthur Grant, D.O. *The Lengthening Shadow of Dr. Andrew Taylor Still.* 2nd ed. Macon, Missouri: (publishers) Mrs. A.G. Hildreth and Mrs. A.E. Vleck, 1942.

Kapit, Wynn, and Lawrence M. Elson. *The Anatomy Coloring Book.* New York, N.Y.: Harper & Row, Publishers, 1977.

Karp, Reba Ann. *Edgar Cayce Encyclopedia of Healing.* New York, N.Y.: Warner Books, Inc., 1986.

Kasseroller, Renato, M.D. *Compendium of Dr. Vodder's Manual Lymph Drainage.* Heidelberg, Germany: Karl F. Haug Verlag, 1998.

Kunz, Jeffrey R.M., M.D., and Asher J. Finkel, M.D. *The American Medical Association Family Medical Guide.* Rev. ed. New York, N.Y.: Random House, Inc., 1982.

Kurz, Ingrid, M.D. *Textbook of Dr. Vodder's Manual Lymph Drainage. Volume 2: Therapy.* 4th ed. Heidelberg, Germany: Karl F. Haug Verlag, 1997.

————. *Textbook of Dr. Vodder's Manual Lymph Drainage. Volume 3: Treatment Manual.* 3rd ed. Brussels, Belgium: Haug International, 1987.

Le Vay, David, M.S., F.R.C.S. *Human Anatomy and Physiology.* (Teach Yourself series). Chicago, Ill.: NTC Publishing Group, 1993.

Marieb, Elaine N., R.N., Ph.D. *Essentials of Human Anatomy and Physiology.* 6th ed. San Francisco, Calif.: Benjamin/Cummings Science Publishing, 2000.

McDonough, James T., Jr., Ph.D. *Stedman's Concise Medical Dictionary*. 2nd ed. Baltimore, Md.: Williams & Wilkins, 1994.

McGarey, William A., M.D. "Edgar Cayce and the Palma Christi." Circulating File: Castor Oil Packs/Palma Christi. Virginia Beach, Va.: A.R.E. Press, 1970, 1992.

————. *The Edgar Cayce Remedies*. New York, N.Y.: Bantam Books, 1983.

————. *The Oil That Heals: A Physician's Successes with Castor Oil Treatments*. Virginia Beach, Va.: A.R.E. Press, 1993.

————, compiler. *Physician's Reference Notebook*. Virginia Beach, Va.: A.R.E. Press, 1999.

McMillan, David, M.A. "Anatomy, Physiology, and Pathology in the Health Readings of Edgar Cayce." (Course). Atlantic University. Virginia Beach, Va., November 2002.

Merck Manual of Medical Information, The. (Home edition). New York, N.Y.: Pocket Books, 1997.

Millard, F.P., D.O. *Applied Anatomy of the Lymphatics*. (Reprint). Pomeroy, Wash.: Health Research, 1964.

Miller, Benjamin, and Claire Keane. *Encyclopedia and Dictionary of Medicine, Nursing, and Allied Health*. 6th ed. Philadelphia, Penn.: W.B. Saunders Company, 1997.

Mindell, Earl, R.Ph.D., Ph.D., and Virginia Hopkins, M.A. *Complete Guide to Natural Cures*. New Canaan, Conn.: Keats Publishing, Inc., 2001.

Nguyen, Sy. *The Human Body*. Paris, France: Editions de La Martinière, 1996.

Pollot, Phillip, L.M.T., C.D.T. *Lymphedema: Finding the Holistic Approach*. Rochester, N.Y.: Phillip Pollot, 2001.

Reilly, Harold J., and Ruth Hagy Brod. *The Edgar Cayce Handbook for Health Through Drugless Therapy*. Rev. ed. Virginia Beach, Va.: A.R.E. Press, 2004.

Rhoades, Rodney, Ph.D., and Richard Pflanzer, Ph.D. *Human Physiology*. Philadelphia, Penn.: Saunders College Publishing, 1989.

Rossiter, Frederick. *Water for Health and Healing*. Riverside, Calif.: H.C. White Publications, 1972.

Solomon, Eldra Pearl. *Introduction to Human Anatomy and Physiology*. Philadelphia, Penn.: W.B. Saunders Company, 1992.

Sugrue, Thomas. *There Is a River: The Story of Edgar Cayce*. Virginia Beach, Va.: A.R.E. Press, 1942, 1945.

Takahashi, Takeo. *Atlas of the Human Body*. New York, N.Y.: Harper Collins Publishers, Inc., 1994.

Tortora, Gerard J., and Sandra Reynolds Grabowski. *Principles of Anatomy and Physiology.* 9th ed. New York, N.Y.: John Wiley & Sons, 2000.

Turner, Gladys Davis, and Mae Gimbert St. Clair, compilers. *Individual Reference File.* Virginia Beach, Va.: A.R.E. Press, 1970, 1976.

Webster's New Explorer Medical Dictionary. Springfield, Mass. Federal Street Press, 1999.

Webster's New World Dictionary. 3rd college ed. New York, N.Y.: Prentice Hall General Reference, 1994.

Weil, Andrew, M.D. *Health and Healing.* Boston, Mass.: Houghton Mifflin Company, 1983.

————. *Natural Health, Natural Medicine: A Comprehensive Manual for Wellness and Self-Care.* Boston, Mass.: Houghton Mifflin Company, 1990.

Weissleder, Horst, and Christian Schuchhardt, eds. *Lymphedema: Diagnosis and Therapy.* 2nd ed. Bonn, Germany: Kagerer Kommunikation, 1997.

Whitfield, Philip, ed. *The Human Body Explained.* New York, N.Y.: Henry Holt and Company, Inc., 1995.

Wittlinger. H. and G. *Textbook of Dr. Vodder's Manual Lymph Drainage: Volume 1: Basic Course.* 5th rev. ed. (English ed.) Brussels, Belgium: Haug International, 1992.

A.R.E. PRESS

The A.R.E. Press publishes books, videos, audiotapes, CDs, and DVDs meant to improve the quality of our readers' lives—personally, professionally, and spiritually. We hope our products support your endeavors to realize your career potential, to enhance your relationships, to improve your health, and to encourage you to make the changes necessary to live a loving, joyful, and fulfilling life.

For more information or to receive a free catalog, call:

800–333–4499

Or write:

A.R.E. Press
215 67th Street
Virginia Beach, VA 23451–2061

ARE PRESS.COM

BAAR PRODUCTS

A.R.E.'s Official Worldwide Exclusive Supplier of Edgar Cayce Health Care Products

Baar Products, Inc., is the official worldwide exclusive supplier of Edgar Cayce health care products. Baar offers a collection of natural products and remedies drawn from the work of Edgar Cayce, considered by many to be the father of modern holistic medicine.

For a complete listing of Cayce-related products, call:

800–269–2502

Or write:

Baar Products, Inc.
P.O. Box 60
Downingtown, PA 19335 U.S.A.
Customer Service and International: 610–873–4591
Fax: 610–873–7945
Web Site: www.baar.com   E–mail: cayce@baar.com

EDGAR CAYCE'S A.R.E.

What Is A.R.E.?

The Association for Research and Enlightenment, Inc., (A.R.E.®) was founded in 1931 to research and make available information on psychic development, dreams, holistic health, meditation, and life after death. As an open-membership research organization, the A.R.E. continues to study and publish such information, to initiate research, and to promote conferences, distance learning, and regional events. Edgar Cayce, the most documented psychic of our time, was the moving force in the establishment of A.R.E.

Who Was Edgar Cayce?

Edgar Cayce (1877–1945) was born on a farm near Hopkinsville, Ky. He was an average individual in most respects. Yet, throughout his life, he manifested one of the most remarkable psychic talents of all time. As a young man, he found that he was able to enter into a self-induced trance state, which enabled him to place his mind in contact with an unlimited source of information. While asleep, he could answer questions or give accurate discourses on any topic. These discourses, more than 14,000 in number, were transcribed as he spoke and are called "readings."

Given the name and location of an individual anywhere in the world, he could correctly describe a person's condition and outline a regimen of treatment. The consistent accuracy of his diagnoses and the effectiveness of the treatments he prescribed made him a medical phenomenon, and he came to be called the "father of holistic medicine."

Eventually, the scope of Cayce's readings expanded to include such subjects as world religions, philosophy, psychology, parapsychology, dreams, history, the missing years of Jesus, ancient civilizations, soul growth, psychic development, prophecy, and reincarnation.

A.R.E. Membership

People from all walks of life have discovered meaningful and life-transforming insights through membership in A.R.E. To learn more about Edgar Cayce's A.R.E. and how membership in the A.R.E. can enhance your life, visit our Web site at EdgarCayce.org, or call us toll-free at 800-333-4499.

Edgar Cayce's A.R.E.
215 67th Street
Virginia Beach, VA 23451–2061

EDGARCAYCE.ORG